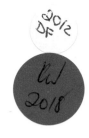

Sex-Selective Abortion in India

SEX-SELECTIVE ABORTION IN INDIA

The Impact on Child Mortality

Mary Elizabeth Shepherd

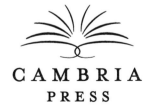

CAMBRIA
PRESS

YOUNGSTOWN, NEW YORK

Library of Congress Cataloging-in-Publication Data
Shepherd, Mary E.

  Sex-selective abortion in India : the impact on child mortality / Mary E. Shepherd.
        p. cm.
     Includes bibliographical references and index.
     ISBN 978-1-934043-69-1 (alk. paper)
     1. Abortion—India. 2.   Sex preselection. 3.   Children—Mortality—India. I. Title.
     [DNLM: 1.   Abortion, Induced—India—Statistics. 2.   Sex Factors—India—Statistics. 3.   Child—India. 4.   Child Mortality—India. 5.   Infant—India. 6.   Morbidity—India—Statistics. 7.   Prejudice—India. 8.   Sex Ratio—India—Statistics. HQ 767.5.I5 S548s 2007]

   HQ767.5.I5S54 2007
   304.6'670954--dc22

2007032711

For my niece,
Sara Anil Rohra Shepherd,
one of the girls represented
among the 1992 births
in Maharashtra.

TABLE OF CONTENTS

LIST OF TABLES

LIST OF FIGURES

List of Figures

LIST OF MAPS

ACKNOWLEDGMENTS

This work could never have come to fruition had it not been for the efforts of the International Institute for Population Sciences in Mumbai and ORC Macro in Calverton, MD for collecting, compiling, and making available publicly the National Family Health Survey data used in this study. Many thanks are due to those who provided thoughtful comments on the work: Dr. Michael Koenig, Dr. Amy Tsui, and Dr. Norma Kanarek of Johns Hopkins University, Dr. Sanjay Mehendale of the National AIDS Research Institute, and Dr. Mona Sharan of the World Bank. The editorial contributions and the patience of the staff at Cambria Press, especially Sharon Berger, are greatly appreciated. Fellowship support was provided by the Department of Population, Family, and Reproductive Health of the Johns Hopkins University Bloomberg School of Public Health.

SEX-SELECTIVE
ABORTION IN INDIA

CHAPTER 1

INTRODUCTION

BACKGROUND AND SIGNIFICANCE

Indian government officials were disappointed by India's poor ranking in the 2002 United Nations Development Report—124th of 173 countries—and the report's criticism of social development issues, focusing particularly on the situation of women and health (Jacob, 2002). The report highlighted the large estimated number of "missing women" in India (Fukuda-Parr, 2002), using the term *Nobel laureate Amartya Sen*, coined to draw attention to the abnormally high age-specific mortality rates of females in many Asian and North African populations (Sen, 1990).

Recent demographic studies indicate that the overall sex ratio in India is a poor indicator of recent trends in the status of women because it is the accumulation of unequal child mortality over the past century (Griffiths, Matthews, & Hinde, 2000; Guillot, 2002; Mayer, 1999). A more specific and dynamic indicator is the sex ratio of young children in India, where the trend in missing females appears to be worsening. Indeed, former Health Minister Sushma Swaraj expressed concern that India is at risk of becoming "a daughterless nation" (Carmichael, 2004).

Provisional data from the 2001 census of India show an increase in the ratio of the number of male to female children since the 1991 census. The ratio of the child population aged 0 to 6 years in 2001 was 107.8 males per 100 females,[1] an increase from the 1991 census ratio of 105.8, representing a deficit of nearly 6 million young girls. This continues the trend observed nationwide from 1961 onward, with a particularly sharp incline evident since 1981, as shown in Figure 1.1 (DasGupta & Bhat, 1997; Registrar General of India, 2001). Although the sharpest declines in the relative number of girls were observed in the more affluent Northern states of Punjab, Haryana, Himachal Pradesh as well as in the Western/Central state of Gujarat, decreases were observed nationwide, with 77% of all districts recording higher male-to-female (M:F) child population ratios in 2001 than in 1991 (Registrar General of India, 2001). Appendix Maps A.1.1 and A.1.2 display the 2001 juvenile sex ratio by district for the rural and urban populations. This reduction in the relative number of female children could be due to a combination of factors: changes in the sex ratio at birth due to the diffusion of sex-selective abortion, an increase in the mortality of female children relative to male children, as well as to data errors such as changes in the census undercount of girls relative to boys (Dyson, 2001).

The availability first of amniocentesis in the late 1970s (Ramanama & Bambawale, 1980 as cited in Ganatra, Hirve, & Rao, 2001) followed by more widespread use of ultrasound in the

Figure 1.1. Sex ratio of the 0- to 6-year-old population, India.

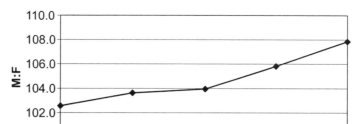

Census year

Sources. DasGupta and Bhatt (1997); and Registrar General of India (2001).

early to mid-1980s to selectively abort female fetuses (Claycraft, 1989) corresponds in time to the sharp decline in the relative number of Indian girls, suggesting that sex-selective abortion is likely to be a substantial contributing factor. As shown in Appendix Figure A.1.1, estimates of the sex ratio at birth in India have increased during the 1990s, especially among higher order births and among births in urban areas to more educated mothers. In an attempt to eliminate the practice of sex-selective abortion, the government of India passed legislation in 1994 banning prenatal sex-determination testing. The Prenatal Diagnostic Techniques (Regulation and Prevention of Misuse) Act of 1994 went into effect in January 1996; however, it has not been enforced effectively. Private ultrasound clinics have proliferated, and mobile clinics have made prenatal sex determination increasingly available in rural areas.

Sen (2003) notes that recent improvements in excess female child mortality have been counterbalanced by "a new female disadvantage—that in natality" (p. 1297). It is not clear, however, the degree to which prenatal and postnatal gender differentials in mortality may be interacting with each other in India. Goodkind (1999) has suggested that it may be unethical to ban sex-selective abortion in part because of the potentially detrimental effect on postnatal female mortality. It may well be that enforcement of the Prenatal Diagnostic Techniques Act in the absence of policy initiatives addressing the potential ensuing increases in female postnatal mortality, will have a deleterious effect on the juvenile sex ratio. Goodkind notes that empirical testing of this potential shift from prenatal to postnatal discrimination has been precluded by limitations in the comparative design of recent research and a lack of appropriate data. Nonetheless, using causal modeling of observational data, it is possible to make substantive analytical inferences about policy alternatives with respect to sex-selective abortion using Demographic and Health Survey (DHS) data (Cole & Hernan, 2002; Pearl, 2001; Robins, Hernan, & Brumback, 2000; Smith, 2003; Winship & Morgan, 1999).

CHAPTER 2

BACKGROUND ON POPULATION SEX RATIO

HUMAN SECONDARY SEX RATIO

The primary sex ratio of sperm in mammals is 1:1, but a higher proportion of fetuses are male, possibly as a result of preferential binding of Y-chromosome sperm to the oocyte. Figure 2.1 shows estimates of the changing sex ratio over the course of gestation (Broer, Weber, & Kaiser, 1977; Kukharenko, 1973).

In mammals, the number of male live births exceeds female live births. For humans, the male proportion of births is expected to be approximately 0.513, or 103–106 male births per 100 female births (United Nations Secretariat, 1998). John Graunt was the first to compile data that showed an excess of male over female births in the 17th century (Petty, 1964, as cited in Campbell, 2001). He noted in 1662, using parish records of births

Figure 2.1. Sex ratio by gestational age.

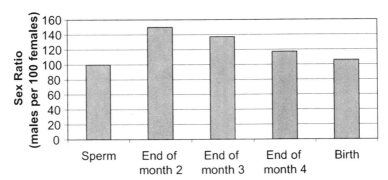

and deaths, that there were more male infants born annually in London than female infants, and he also documented that more male infants died during the 1st year of life than female infants.

It has been thought that timing of insemination affects the primary sex ratio (sex ratio of conceptions) and thus subsequently the sex ratio of births. Fertilization early in the cycle is theorized to yield a greater proportion of male fetuses, and has been proposed as an explanation for increased sex ratio at birth during and after the World Wars. Contrary to this theory, in a multicenter, prospective study of pregnancies among women using natural family planning, Gray et al. (1998), analyzed data from diaries of coitus and menses and found that the sex ratio among 947 singleton births did not vary consistently or significantly with the estimated timing of insemination relative to the day of ovulation, or with the estimated length of the follicular phase.

A lower sex ratio at birth was found among women with a vegetarian diet in a relatively small study of several thousand nonvegetarian and several hundred vegetarian women (Hudson & Buckley, 2000). However, these results were not replicated in a nationally representative sample of births from India that included a large number of both vegetarian and nonvegetarian women (Arnold & Roy, 2001). Similarly, parental age gap has been hypothesized as a causal factor in altered sex ratio at birth (Manning, Anderton, & Shutt, 1997), but no association was found between the difference in parents' ages and sex ratio at birth when very large national samples were analyzed (Arnold et al., 1997) or in a large sample from northern Italy (Astolfi & Zonta, 1999).

There is some evidence that acute psychological stress may result in a lower sex ratio: In Slovenia 6 to 9 months after the 1991 war, a significant decrease in the sex ratio at birth was detected (Zorn, Sucur, Stare, & Meden-Vrtovec, 2002). The investigators analyzed the motility of sperm over time among men with baseline normal sperm levels from fertility clinic records and found a decline in sperm mobility during the time of the war. A decline in the sex ratio at birth was found after the earthquake in Kobe, Japan (Fukuda, Fukuda, Shimizu, & Moller, 1998). A Kurdish city in Iran had a decline in the sex ratio at birth following a mustard gas attack (Saadat, 2006). James' hypothesis, that parental hormone levels around the time of conception affect the sex of the fetus, provide a mechanism for these study findings (James, 2004).

Recent studies have examined how perinatal viral infections may differentially affect male and female fetuses. In a study of the vertical transmission of human immunodeficiency virus (HIV) in Malawi, Taha et al. (2005) found that girls were more likely to be born infected (12.6%) than boys (6.3%). The M:F sex ratio at birth, however, was less than one (0.968) for this study population of HIV-infected women, indicating an adverse in utero effect on males. Similarly, infant girls were twice as likely to be born with hepatitis C virus as boys in two recent studies (European Paediatric Hepatitis C Virus Network, 2005; Mast et al., 2005). Beasley (2005) noted the low sex ratio at birth in one of the studies, and suggested that excess male mortality in utero is more likely than a higher infection rate among female infants. The *opposite* effect has been posited as an explanation for the skewed sex ratio at birth in many countries where hepatitis B virus (HBV) infections are prevalent. Oster (2005) has estimated that as much as 75% of the "missing females" in China and 20% of those in India can be accounted for by differential in utero mortality of female offspring of HBV-infected women. Das Gupta (2005) countered that the data showing the variability of sex ratio at birth by parity and by the sex composition of older siblings do not support this viral hypothesis. Beasley (2005) points out that males of all ages have slightly higher HBV infection rates than females, poorer immune responses to HBV vaccination, and a higher incidence of sequelae of infection such as chronic hepatitis, cirrhosis, and hepatocellular carcinoma; thus, it is unlikely that females would have higher in utero mortality.

SEX RATIO OF THE POPULATION IN INDIA

Although males are more vulnerable biologically in the perinatal and infant periods, in parts of South and East Asia and North Africa young females face mortality disadvantages based on social and behavioral factors (Arnold, 1992; Sen 1992; Waldron, 1987). The main pathway to excess female mortality is likely to be differential allocation of household resources to male and female children (Arnold, 1992; Basu, 1989; Bourne & Walker, 1991; Chen, Huq, & D'Souza, 1981; Das Gupta, 1987; Hill & Upchurch, 1995; Miller, 1989).

India has had a long-standing imbalance in the population sex ratio favoring males. Indeed, the first census of India administered by the British in 1872 revealed a severe deficit of women (Miller, 1981). The M:F sex ratio has shown an increase of 1% at each subsequent decennial census over the course of the 20th century (Registrar General of India, 1995, as cited in Mayer, 1999).

Recent demographic studies have focused on the long-term effects of historical changes in levels of mortality and changing gender differentials in mortality on the current population sex ratio. Analyzing national-level data, Mayer (1999) concluded that the secular increase in the M:F sex ratio in India is due to gender differentials in the rate of demographic transition. Health and nutritional status of children has improved at a slightly faster pace for males than females resulting over a long time period in increasing secular trends in the sex ratio. The increase is an artifact of long-term improvements in life expectancy leading to population increase, which occurs at a different rate for girls and boys. Griffiths, Matthews, & Hinde (2000) used a simulation approach to show that excess female mortality persisting over the long-term can continue to produce an increase in the male-to-female population sex ratios, even when excess female mortality is in decline. Guillot (2002) cautions against using the overall population sex ratio as a proxy for sex differentials in mortality, and estimates that excess female mortality peaked around 1968, and has been declining since then. The atypically masculine sex ratios found in the 1971 and 1991 censuses are thought to be attributable to differential census undercount of females (Dyson, 2001; Guillot, 2002).

This work does not address the complex issue of population sex ratios, but focuses on sex ratio at birth and sex differentials in under-five mortality, which are not subject to long-term cohort effects or to the effects of sex-specific migration patterns.

DETERMINANTS OF SON PREFERENCE

Economic Factors

Bardhan (1974) hypothesized that it is current economic forces that determine the social value of women and that female agricultural labor force participation can explain geographic variability in gender mortality differentials in India. In the northern areas where wheat is the primary crop, plow agriculture, and more recently mechanized agriculture, preclude women's participation in the production process. In the south of India, which has been characterized by narrower gender differentials in mortality, rice cultivation is common, which is a labor-intensive process and fully utilizes the labor of women. Miller (1981) found a correlation between female labor force participation and juvenile sex ratios in the 1961 census at the district level, and Kishor (1993) found a similar relationship with sex ratios of child mortality. Gupta and Attari (1994) added to the evidence by noting that changes in female labor participation were correlated with changes in the sex ratio. Women's workforce participation has declined over the course of the 20th century from a high of 34% in 1911 to a low of 20% in 1981, whereas the ratio of planted wheat to rice has increased, along with the secular increase in the sex ratio (Mayer, 1999).

Cultural Factors

Marvin Harris (1993) theorized that social relations characterized by male dominance in societies, such as that of the upper Gangetic plain, developed from the reliance on draught-animal agriculture. In contrast to hoe agriculture, which predominated in West Africa, body strength was needed to produce efficiently from the hard-packed soil, which required deep plowing with traction animals after the dry season. Plow agriculture led to a high population density and shortages of arable land, which in turn resulted in lower value of labor and of the reproductive capacities of women (Goody, 1973; 1976). Men's control over traction animals, which also were the means of land transport, led to dominance in trade and commerce, government administration, and state religions. Over the long term, practices initially induced by material forces developed into entrenched cultural norms.

Dyson and Moore (1983) theorized that it is not strictly economic forces that determine the wide gap between male and female survival in northern India but cultural forces in the form of marriage and kinship patterns. Exogamous marriage and kinship—marrying out of the natal village and out of the family—is a practice common in North India (Aryan) that decreases women's autonomy and their social value. The flow of resources is culturally dictated to be from the bride's family to the groom's family, which manifests as dowry payments and often gifts throughout the life course as well. Marriage rules dictate that a woman must marry into a higher caste family (hypergamy). Thus, daughters are a means of enhancing social status; families negotiate a higher status for themselves by marrying their daughters into a higher caste family. Women are precluded from inheritance of land. In the south of India (Dravidian), consanguinity, or cross-cousin marriage, is more common. Women tend to marry within their natal villages and maintain close social and economic ties with their natal family. There is greater status equality between wife-givers and wife-takers, and a woman may marry into a lower caste family.

The north/south dichotomy has been criticized by Caldwell and Caldwell (1990), who consider the appropriate distinction to be between the "heartland of an ancient peasant civilization and its periphery" (p. 11). Rather than a static north/south geographic divide, Berreman (1993) describes an Indo-Aryan "core," and sociopolitical "periphery." The dominant Hindu ethos characteristic of the core Indo-Aryan culture includes a strong age and gender hierarchy. This dominant culture spread from the upper Gangetic plain of the northeast, assimilating local languages and cultural practices to varying degrees. Regions that are geographically proximate to the core yet remain peripheral are characterized either by a high concentration of tribal populations or by regions that historically resisted the Indo-Aryan expansion, such as the powerful Magadh kingdom in the present-day state of Bihar, which had strong Buddhist, Jainist, and other sectarian influences.

Female Literacy

Studies of the effects of female literacy in the population and mother's level of education on excess female child mortality have had conflicting results. Mayer (1999) analyzed secular trends in female literacy and trends in the population sex ratio at the national level in India from 1911 to 1991, finding that as female literacy increased, the relative number of females decreased.

Several studies in India have found that relative mortality of girls is lower among mothers with more education (Bourne & Walker, 1991; Rosenzweig & Schultz, 1982; Simmons, Smucker, Bernstein, & Jensen, 1982), and Murthi, Guio, & Dreze (1995) found at the district level that female literacy was associated with lower excess female child mortality, which did not vary by geographic (North/South) region. Male literacy was associated with greater excess female child mortality at the district level due to greater reductions in mortality for boys than for girls. Das Gupta (1987), on the other hand, found that in Punjab excess female mortality was higher among daughters of women with some education than among those of women with no education. These discrepant findings may result from the context-dependent social and behavioral effects of female literacy.

Physical and Social Security
Oldenburg (1992) studied the correlation between violence and population sex ratios in Uttar Pradesh, finding a correlation between high M:F sex ratios and murder rates at the district level. He hypothesized that variability in sex ratio by region can be accounted for by the level of violence and by the need for males in the family for day-to-day protection and security as well as by physical support in family and village affairs.

In a nationwide study, Dreze and Khera (2000) found that the population sex ratio was the strongest predictor of murder rates at the district level. Most murders were committed by young men, and the majority were disputes over property or over women. To sort out the direction of causality, a two-stage analysis was performed using female labor force participation as an instrumental variable for sex ratio. If Oldenburg's hypothesis

that level of violence influences the sex ratio was correct, and if
the instrument was appropriately specified, then the statistical
correlation between sex ratio and murder rate should disappear
in the two-stage model, which it does not. This study indicates
that causality may in fact be from masculine population to level
of violence, or more likely, that both are jointly influenced by
an unobserved societal factor, such as the degree of patriarchal
norms.

Cain (1981, 1986) suggested that son preference stems from
the need for insurance against risk, which, in the social and cultural context of South Asia, only sons are entitled to provide.
He examined the means of support, living arrangements, and
quality of life of elderly men and women in 343 households in
Bangladesh and in 320 households in India. Poverty, divorce,
and widowhood were more likely among women without a
mature son, although the effects in India were not as severe as
in Bangladesh due to greater availability of alternative living
arrangements.

PRENATAL CONSEQUENCES OF SON PREFERENCE

Differential Stopping Behavior

Sex ratio at birth within families may be affected by differential
stopping behavior; that is, families continue to bear children
until they reach the desired sex composition of offspring.
In the context of son preference, families who initially have
more daughters will continue to bear children until the desired
number of sons are born, resulting in both a higher family size
and skewed sex ratios of children ever born within families. A
family that has sons early and stops childbearing will have a

high proportion of sons, whereas a family that has sons later will have a lower proportion of sons, even though preference for sons may be the same in both families. Clark (2000) used the 1992–1993 National Family Health Survey (NFHS) data to determine if differential stopping behavior was occurring in India. She compared the ideal and the actual proportion of sons within families and identified characteristics associated with each. As confirmed by her analysis, without controlling for family size, the actual proportion of sons should not be associated with family characteristics in the absence of prenatal sex selection (which was not as widespread by the early 1990s). The ideal proportion of sons was associated with lack of formal education, scheduled caste status, rural residence, and negatively associated with Christian religion and with living in South India. Increasing family size had the opposite effect on ideal and actual proportion of sons: The actual proportion of sons decreased, whereas the ideal proportion increased, indicating that families are not able to meet their ideal number of sons without increasing family size. Restricting the analysis to completed families only and controlling for family size, the actual proportion of sons was significantly associated with lack of formal education, lower caste status, rural residence, Hindu and Muslim religions, and with living in northern and eastern India, indicating that families with those characteristics are more likely to practice differential stopping behavior as a strategy to achieve their desired number of sons.

Sex-Selective Abortion

Abortion has been legal in India since the Medical Termination of Pregnancy Act was passed in 1971. Using chorionic villi sampling, the sex of a fetus can be known as early as 8–10 weeks of gestation, but this method is expensive and is not widely available in India. Amniocentesis was the first method available in India in the 1970s and can detect the sex of a fetus as early as 15–17 weeks, but again is expensive and requires special equipment. Sonography or an ultrasound exam is the least invasive and least expensive method and is nearly 100% accurate by 20 weeks of gestation, but it cannot determine the sex of the fetus until the second trimester. This is the most widely used method for prenatal sex determination in India, although it is technically illegal since the 1994 passage of the Prenatal Diagnostic Techniques (Regulation and Prevention of Misuse) Act. Mobile ultrasound equipment has made sex determination testing available even in remote rural areas. Until recently, sex-selective abortion has been accepted as a means of achieving the desired family composition, based on the fundamental belief in the necessity of having sons and in a couple's right to have them (Arnold, Kishor, & Roy, 2002).

Estimates of the number of sex-selective abortions annually in India range from a minimum of 106,000 based on survey self-reports of prenatal ultrasound and of induced abortion incidence (Arnold et al., 2002) to a conservative estimate of 500,000 based on sex ratio at birth data from a national sample of over 1 million households (Jha et al., 2006). Since prenatal sex determination testing and sex-selective abortion are illegal, they are likely to be severely underreported; thus, estimates based on self-report are likely to be considerably lower than the actual number.

Arnold et al. (2002) found an increase in the sex ratio at birth in the 5 years prior to NFHS-2 (1998–1999) compared to

NFHS-1 (1992–1993) from 105.1 to 106.9, and 16 of 26 states had ratios of 107 or higher in the latter period. Similarly, the sex ratio at birth following an induced abortion in the states of Gujarat, Haryana, and Punjab was extremely elevated, 158.0, whereas in the southern states of Andhra Pradesh, Karnataka, Kerala, and Tamil Nadu it was 107.9; and among mothers who reported receiving an ultrasound, the sex ratio at birth was 128.7 in Gujarat, Haryana, and Punjab and 100.3 in the southern states.

Ganatra, Hirve, and Rao (2001) found in a study of 1,409 rural women in Maharashtra during the period from 1996–1998 that 18% of abortions were obtained for the purpose of sex-selection. Since there are an estimated 4–5 million abortions in India each year, that raises considerably the estimated number of sex-selective abortions per year to 700,000–900,000 compared to the 106,000 estimated by Arnold et al. (2002) and to the 500,000 estimated by Jha et al. (2006). Several hospital-based studies in Punjab have investigated the sex ratio at birth (Booth, Verma, & Beri, 1994; Sachar et al., 1990), showing a high ratio in 1988 of 121.8 and an increase over the 1980s from 107 in 1982 to 132 in 1993. Factors associated with use of fetal sex determination (Booth et al., 1994) included income, education, and sex composition of older siblings. Use increased with increasing monthly income and was common (63%) among those families with no sons and one or more daughters. As the level of the mother's education increased, so did use of sex determination testing.

Retherford and Roy (2003) used data from NFHS-1 and NFHS-2 to analyze factors related to the sex ratio at birth as an indicator of sex-selective abortion. The most significant predictor was a composite of birth order and the number of older living sons. The estimated sex ratio at birth was significantly higher among second-order births with no surviving older brothers (110) and among third-order births with no surviving older brothers (113); however, this was only the case for births reported in NFHS-2 (1984–1998). Also in NFHS-2, births to women who had completed middle school or higher were more likely to be male (112), as were births to mothers of religions other than Hindu or Muslim (115) and births to women with greater media exposure (112). Among births reported in NFHS-1 (1978–1992), urban residents had a significantly elevated sex ratio at birth (110), and Muslims had a significantly lower sex ratio at birth (102). These authors also found limited evidence of the selective abortion of boys in particular states among third-order births to women with two living sons: In NFHS-1, sex ratios at birth were 99 in Punjab, 73 in Delhi, and 93 in Maharashtra, and in NFHS-2, they were 90, 87, and 87, respectively.

A recent study by Jha et al. (2006), utilizing birth history data from the 1998 Special Fertility and Mortality Survey of 1.1 million households nationwide, found that among 133,738 births in 1997, the sex ratio for second births when the preceding child was a girl was 132, compared to 90.7 if the preceding child was a boy. Similarly, for third births, when the previous two children were girls the sex ratio was 139 and when they were boys—85.0. Mothers with a grade 10 or higher level of education had a sex ratio of 146 for the second birth when the first child was a girl; however, no differences were found by religion. By geographic location, the highest sex ratios were found in the North, in the state of Punjab, the city of Delhi, and the states of Bihar, Haryana, Gujarat, Rajasthan, and Uttar Pradesh.

POSTNATAL CONSEQUENCES OF SON PREFERENCE

Excess Female Infant Mortality

Khanna, Kumar, Vaghela, Sreenivas, and Puliyel (2003) carried out a community-based study of infant deaths in three economically deprived areas on the outskirts of Delhi, India. Verbal autopsy data collected on 442 infant deaths from 1997 to 2001 were analyzed to determine if there was a gender differential in preventable infant mortality. There were 7,012 births during the study period, with a sex ratio at birth of 115 boys per 100 girls. For girls, the infant mortality rate was 1.3 times higher than for boys. Diarrhea was the most common cause of death (21%), followed by birth asphyxia (14%), immaturity (12%), acute respiratory infection (11%), and unexplained cause (10%). Girls were found to have significantly higher mortality rates than boys for diarrhea and unexplained deaths, whereas boys did not have significantly higher infant mortality rates within any of the cause-of-death categories. For causes of infant death that were less treatable or preventable, such as birth asphyxia, immaturity, septicemia, and congenital anomalies, no differences were found in mortality rates by gender. The rate of "unexplained death" was 3.5 times higher in girls than boys. Half of the 44 unexplained deaths occurred in the first month of life, and 19 of those 22 unexplained neonatal deaths occurred among girls. For preventable and treatable diarrheal disease, the cause-specific mortality was found to be 2.3 times higher among female infants than male infants.

Excess Female Under-5 Mortality

Das Gupta (1987) studied discrimination against girls at the household level in rural Punjab, finding that sex bias within the

family is not generalized, but is strategically targeted toward
daughters of higher birth order and specifically toward those
with at least one older sister. On average women reported that
their ideal family composition consisted of one to two sons
and zero to one daughter. The lowest mortality rate was found
among boys with no older brothers, whereas boys with one or
more older brothers had a child mortality rate slightly higher
than that of first-born girls. These patterns suggest that family-
building strategies lead parents to differentially allocate environmental and care inputs to their sons and daughters according
to their position in and importance to the family. This pattern
was even more pronounced among the younger mothers, where
daughters with an older sister had 71% higher child mortality,
a surprising finding at the time given that the younger women
had much higher levels of education and that their overall child
mortality levels were substantially lower. This finding was
attributed to the smaller family size among the younger, more
educated women who are under greater pressure to limit their
family to a single daughter, so they can still have the desired
one to two sons. Das Gupta points out that educated women are
better able to control both fertility and mortality and are thus
better able to match their achieved and desired family sex composition by selectively allocating care to the wanted children.
Examination by socioeconomic status showed that overall child
mortality varied by land ownership, but the pattern of selective
neglect did not. Second-born daughters of both landed and landless parents had 50% higher mortality than other children.

Several studies have found that the beneficial effect of female
labor force participation on gender differentials in child mortality is magnified in the northern regions, where the cultural

context is less favorable to women (Agnihotri, Palmer-Jones, & Parikh, 2002; Kishor, 1993). Agnihotri et al. italicized. found an interaction between female labor force participation and cultural patterns on child sex ratios in a district-level analysis of 1981 census data. Greater levels of female labor force participation were associated with less masculine juvenile sex ratios, and in North India, the effect was more pronounced than in southern India. Similarly, Kishor (1993) found that patrilocal exogamy was the strongest predictor of high excess female child mortality and that the effect was even stronger where female labor force participation was the lowest. This suggests that increasing the economic worth of females where their cultural worth is the lowest will be more effective in narrowing gender differentials in child mortality than increasing their economic worth where their cultural worth is higher. Rice cultivation was associated with narrower gaps in gender differentials even after the analysis controlled for women's labor force participation, contrary to the theory that women's status is higher in South India due to greater demand for female labor in rice cultivation.

Differential Nutrition and Health Care

To fill the gap in the literature on factors affecting gender differentials in morbidity rather than mortality in India, Pande (2003) investigated the impact of family composition on gender differentials in nutritional status and immunization status among surviving children under age 5 in rural India using data from the NFHS-1 survey. The presence of older siblings of the same gender was found to adversely affect nutritional status for daughters and vaccination coverage for sons, indicating that parents allocate resources in a manner that favors a family with balanced gender composition of children. Having an older same-sex sibling had a statistically significant impact on severe stunting of girls but not boys. Boys with two or more older brothers were, however, significantly less likely to be immunized than first-born sons, a finding not replicated among the girls. Boys in families with two or more older sisters and no older brothers enjoyed particular health advantages, being significantly more likely to be immunized and marginally less likely to be stunted than boys with no older siblings.

Sex differentials in childhood feeding, health care, and nutritional status over the decade of the 1990s in India were investigated using data from the two NFHS surveys (Mishra, Roy, & Rutherford, 2004). Their analyses were stratified by both birth order and the number of older living sons to test the hypothesis that patterns of gender discrimination are consistent with family building strategies resulting in at least one daughter and one or more sons. Although third-born sons were less likely to be exclusively breastfed at 6–9 months compared to daughters with two older brothers, no consistent and clear pattern of gender discrimination was observed across all birth orders. Similarly, boys of birth order 3 with two older sisters were more likely to be fully immunized than girls with two older sisters. The manifestation of gender discrimination particularly among children of birth order 3 may arise because the total fertility rate in India is close to 3; thus, the third-born child is of particular importance for achieving the desired family composition. Treatment-seeking behavior for acute respiratory infections and for diarrhea showed a preference for sons that weakened as the number of older living sons increased, with the strongest pattern at birth order 3. These patterns were more pronounced in the Northern states than the Southern states. Among families with no older girls in the South, full immunization and treatment seeking for illness among higher birth order children tended to favor girls rather than boys. Among higher birth order children, the occurrence of stunting and below normal weight showed a clear pattern of discrimination against girls in families where boys were in short supply and discrimination against boys in families where girls were scarce. However, measures of wasting and anemia showed no such pattern. These findings, similar to those of Pande (2003), underscore the need to specify the family composition of older siblings in studies of gender discrimination in children's nutritional status, since countervailing trends may cancel out each effect in aggregate analyses.

Das Gupta (1987) examined gender differentials in expenditures for clothing and medicine and in food allocation in Punjab. The study revealed that 2.3 times more was spent on medicines for boys than girls under the age of 24 months, and 1.4 times more was spent on boys' clothing than girls' clothing. Differentials in food consumption were less marked. Girls under 24 months received 32% more cereals and 2% more sugar than boys, whereas boys received 22% more fat and 9% more milk than girls. Children of landless parents tended to have a greater gender differential in clothing, medicine, and fat allocation than did the children of landed parents but more equal distribution of cereals and overall calories, indicating that scarce resources and expensive commodities are allocated somewhat more carefully in these poorer families.

A hospital-based study found that among admitted children, girls were less likely to be in the newborn or infant age groups, to be of the Sikh religion, or to live far away than were boys, suggesting that these factors may be significant risk factors for denied access to medical care for girls living in Punjab, India (Booth & Verma, 1992). The study did not take into account that male infants and neonates may have worse health for biological reasons that lead to hospitalization.

CHANGES IN SON PREFERENCE
AS FERTILITY DECLINES

Das Gupta and Bhat (1997) explored the relationship at the population level between fertility decline and increasing manifestations of sex bias in India. They identified two countervailing effects of declining fertility on sex bias, which they call the "parity effect" and the "intensification effect" (p. 307). The parity effect refers to the indirect effect that fertility decline has on excess female mortality by reducing the proportion of births that are higher parity births. Since excess female mortality in South Asia is concentrated among higher parity births, fertility decline would be expected to result in a decrease in excess female mortality by changing the distribution of births by parity. The intensification effect refers to the increase in excess female mortality at a given parity as fertility declines, as has been observed in other societies with a strong preference for sons, namely China and South Korea. This effect results from a more rapid decline in the number of wanted children than in the number of wanted sons. "The difference in speed of these two trajectories narrows the space left for daughters" (p. 307). Using data from the Khanna Study in Punjab, Das Gupta and Bhat modeled the effect of a change in the parity distribution of births on excess female child mortality by applying the parity-specific child mortality rates observed to a low-fertility population and noted that it would result in a drop from 9% excess female mortality to 0%. Then, keeping fertility levels at a constant low level, they applied the parity-specific child mortality rates observed among families in Khanna with three or fewer children to model the intensification of male bias and noted a 25% increase in excess female child mortality. Thus, it appears in the Khanna region that the intensification of male bias outweighs the parity effect, resulting in a net increase in excess female child mortality of 25% − 9% = 16%. The authors estimated that over the decade from 1981 to 1991, there were 4.2 million excess female postnatal deaths and more than 1 million sex-selective abortions, or approximately four postnatal excess female deaths for each sex-selective abortion. In terms of the effect of sex discrimination on overall fertility and mortality levels, the estimated levels of sex-selective abortion amount to less than 0.5% of all births and are too low to contribute much to declines in total fertility. On the contrary, the excess mortality of girls does increase overall child mortality considerably, with the excess mortality from 1981 to 1991 alone constituting a child mortality rate of 46 per 1,000 live female births.

In a similar investigation, Basu (1999) explored the trend of increasing sex bias that has accompanied fertility transition in India. She observed that a convergence has taken the place of the North and South gender and fertility regimes as well as a convergence across classes. In the North there is evidence of a rapid pace of fertility decline and a decrease in the extreme gender differentials in postnatal mortality that maintained in the past, whereas in the South there is evidence of an increasing gap between female and male child mortality levels along with moderate to low fertility. She draws on anthropological studies carried out in

Tamil Nadu that suggest that it is the upwardly mobile classes that are practicing the greatest gender discrimination. The changing aspirations brought by modern education, increased mobility, and mass media, largely favoring consumerism, have not been matched by enhanced economic opportunities. For many families, manipulating the gender composition of offspring has become a means of furthering upward mobility, economically and socially. The practice of Northern cultural traditions, such as dowry and *exogamy* (marrying out of the village or kinship network), has increased over time in the South, as has *hypergamy*, where a bride can only marry up to a higher caste and/or higher social status groom. Thus, having a daughter is a means of upward social mobility, whereas having a son is a means of upward economic mobility through receipt of dowry payment.

Bhat and Zavier (2003) recently refuted the hypothesis of Das Gupta and Bhat (1997) that, as fertility declines, gender preferences for sons intensify. They analyzed individual-level data on preferred number of sons and daughters reported by women in northern India in NFHS-1 and NFHS-2 and showed that, after controlling for confounding factors, the proportion of women preferring more sons than daughters and the proportion of their children that women preferred to be sons declined as the ideal family size declined. Indeed, the authors show that this decline is faster than the decline in the preferred number or proportion of girls. Factors independently associated with greater son preference included: greater ideal family size and Hindu and Sikh religions, whereas factors associated with less son preference included: urban residence, exposure to mass media, higher level of education, and scheduled tribe membership. The incongruity of these findings with the secular rise in the juvenile sex ratio over time is explained as a change in the ability of parents to realize sex preferences. With the desire for sons declining at a faster rate than the desire for daughters, the gap between the two narrows over time, but a gap still remains, with sons preferred over daughters. Sixty percent of the unwanted births in the year preceding the NFHS-2 survey were girls. The diffusion of sex-selective technology, allowing parents greater ability to realize their heretofore latent preferences, has increased the manifestation of sex bias over time. The *actual* sex composition of children in the family is converging upon the *desired* composition over time. The moral and emotional cost of an abortion is lower than that of infanticide or neglect of a living child, so even those parents who would not be able to directly or indirectly eliminate their daughters are able to opt for sex-selective abortion; thus, preferences are more attainable.

SUBSTITUTION HYPOTHESIS

As has been shown in China and South Korea, a consequence of fertility decline in the context of male preference is an increasing sex ratio at birth (Park & Cho, 1995). Korea has experienced a concurrent increase in the survival of girls relative to boys; in other words, fewer girls are born, but those that are born appear to be more likely to survive (DasGupta & Bhat, 1997; Goodkind, 1996). China, however, still has higher female infant mortality relative to males but may be a special case due to the strictly enforced one-child policy. Sex-selective abortion thus appears to serve as a substitute for female child mortality in Korea but not in China. The relationship between the sex ratio at birth and the sex ratio of child mortality is not clear in India, where sex-selective abortion may be substituting for, or adding to, female infant and female child mortality. The evidence of an accelerating increase in the M:F sex ratio of the juvenile population after the introduction of inexpensive fetal sex determination technologies would support the theory that sex-selective abortion is an additive to, rather than a substitute for, infant and child mortality in India.

Goodkind (1996) assessed data from several East Asian countries for evidence that prenatal sex selection was substituting for, rather than adding to, postnatal sex preference strategies. Goodkind used vital registration data to examine secular trends in the sex ratio at birth and the sex ratio of infant and child deaths over recent decades in three East Asian countries undergoing fertility transitions: South Korea, China, and Taiwan. The data from Taiwan were found not to meet the two conditions necessary for testing the validity of the substitution hypothesis at the aggregate level: evidence of discrimination against daughters in the form of abnormally low male-to-female ratios of infant and early childhood mortality, followed by a sharp rise in the male-to-female sex ratio at birth after prenatal sex determination testing became available; the observation of a subsequent rise in the male-to-female ratios of infant and child death rates would support the substitution hypothesis. By the mid-1960s, well before fetal sex-testing technology became available, the relative mortality of girls had improved in Taiwan, even though the levels of infant and child mortality still remained quite high. Although Taiwan's experience is not appropriate for testing the substitution hypothesis, it is interesting to note that the sex ratio at birth had increased to 109.5 by 1990, indicating that sex-selective abortion may be acceptable there, whereas neglect of female children may not be.

Data from Korea show evidence of substantial discrimination against female infants and young girls prior to the 1980s in the form of male-to-female child mortality sex ratios well below 1.0. A rise in the male-to-female sex ratio at birth occurred during the 1980s, reaching 114 by 1990, accompanied by an increase in the male-to-female sex ratio of infant and child mortality to 1.04 and 1.16, respectively. These data support the substitution of prenatal for postnatal discrimination against girls in Korea. On the other hand, China experienced a similar increase in the male-to-female sex ratio at birth during the 1980s but no concurrent increase in the postnatal sex ratio of mortality was observed. In China, prenatal and postnatal sex preference strategies appear to be additive to, rather than substitutes for, each other. China implemented a strict one-child policy in 1979, which puts extreme pressure on families to have their one child be the gender that will be of the most long-term benefit to the family.

Banister and Hill (2004) examined secular trends in mortality by sex in China using the growth balance method and found that following the political and economic reforms of the late 1970s and the implementation of the one-child policy in 1979, overall mortality of 1- to 4-year-old children declined, male infant mortality declined, and female infant mortality rose. From 1949–1977 the long-standing shortage of girls in China improved, but from 1978 to the present, there has been a steady increase in the male-to-female ratio of the juvenile population. The sex ratio among 0- to 4-year-old children at the end of the 1990s was 120 males per 100 females. Banister found that in China, females are less likely than males to survive until the age of 3; then after age 3, they are just as likely to survive as boys.

INFANT AND CHILD MORTALITY

Of the 10.8 million deaths among children under the age of 5 years in 2000, 34% occurred in South Asia (Black, Morris, & Bryce, 2003). Although India had the highest number of child deaths, the country ranked 54th highest by mortality rate. The leading contributors to child mortality are respiratory ailments and infectious and gastro-intestinal diseases, all of which are often exacerbated by underlying malnutrition. A recent systematic review of studies published since 1980 estimated that 52% of under-age-5 mortality in South Asia was attributable to neonatal and "other" causes, 23% to pneumonia, 23% to diarrhea, 1% to measles, and <1% to malaria (Morris, Black, & Tomaskovic, 2003).

WANTEDNESS

There have been few studies outside of the developed countries investigating the prenatal and postnatal consequences of pregnancy intention status. Marston and Cleland (2003) analyzed DHS data for Bolivia, Egypt, Kenya, Peru, and the Philippines to determine if births reported as having been unwanted at conception had worse outcomes in terms of antenatal care, supervised delivery, full vaccination, and stunting. Controlling for birth order and sociodemographic factors, unwanted births were significantly less likely to receive antenatal care in Peru and the Philippines, to have a supervised delivery in Peru, and to be fully vaccinated by age 12 months in Peru and Kenya. Stunting among those under age 5 was significantly more likely among unwanted births only in Peru. Overall, unwanted status did not have a consistent impact across outcomes or across countries, except for Peru, where traditional methods of contraception predominate.

In contrast, another study of DHS data found stunting in toddlers to be related to maternal pregnancy intention status in Bolivia (Shapiro-Mendoza, Selwyn, Smith, & Sanderson, 2005). Children 12–35 months of age from unwanted pregnancies (33% of the sample) and mistimed pregnancies (21% of the sample) were both found to have a 30% greater risk of stunting than children from intended pregnancies. The study controlled for maternal education, birth order, type of toilet facility, and health service use. No differences were found in stunting among infants. Paternal pregnancy intention was also analyzed in this study and found to contribute additional risk of stunting above that conferred by maternal pregnancy intention.

Montgomery, Lloyd, Hewett, and Heuveline (1997) analyzed DHS data from five countries from 1987–1993 and found a weak association of unwanted fertility with mortality in Egypt, the Philippines, and Thailand, and the analysis found an association between unwanted fertility and stunting in the Dominican Republic. Small negative effects of having unwanted children in the family were found on educational attainment of siblings in the Dominican Republic, the Philippines, and Thailand.

CHAPTER 3

CONCEPTUAL FRAMEWORK

Agnihotri 1999 has suggested that a useful theoretical framework for the study of gender disparities is provided by the juxtaposition of Amartya Sen's entitlements framework, capabilities approach, and the cooperative-conflict model of intra-household resource allocation. Although, there are disagreements about the relative impact of cultural factors and economic factors on son preference in India, the evidence indicates that the consequence is a differential allocation of resources, such as calories, nutrients, and health care, within the household. Higher mortality of daughters as a result of unequal access to resources can be seen as an entitlement failure (Sen, 1981). This framework accounts for the paradox of higher relative mortality of girls in the most prosperous regions of India and in wealthier households, where there is not a general scarcity of resources (Das Gupta, 1987). The process by which lack of access to resources translates into higher mortality depends upon the context, an issue addressed by the capabilities approach (Sen, 1985).

The overall study framework is shown in Figure 3.1. Son preference can be understood as a deficit of entitlement for females. The determinants of son preference include long-standing cultural norms, gender-based division of labor, lack of female literacy, and the adoption of the custom of dowry. Effects of modernization, such as mass media exposure, education, and physical mobility, may be driving aspirations for consumer goods without providing adequate opportunities to achieve those desires through employment, making dowry an increasingly important means of acquiring financial mobility (Basu, 1999). Son preference is magnified by the presence of one or more older sisters who have exhausted the family's limited role for daughters. Similarly, son preference is dampened by the presence of two or more older brothers.

The consequences of son preference may manifest either before or after birth. Prenatal consequences are differential stopping behavior, which is the adoption of stopping rules to limit childbearing based on the presence of an adequate number of sons, and sex-selective abortion. Postnatal consequences are presented in terms of the Mosley and Chen (1984) proximate determinants of child mortality framework for analyzing the social and biological determinants of child mortality, shown in an abbreviated and modified form in Figure 3.1. The Mosley and Chen framework takes into account the multifactorial causal nature of child mortality in low-resource countries. The death of a child is modeled as the cumulative consequence of a series of biological insults rather than the outcome of a single event or cause. Frailty and vulnerability increase with multiple episodes

Figure 3.1. Overall conceptual framework for the study.

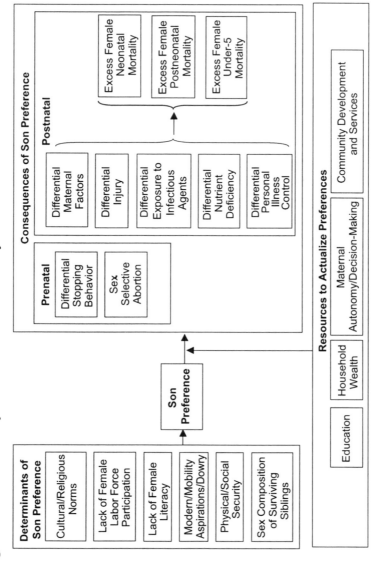

of inadequately treated infection combined with deficiencies of micronutrients and/or macronutrients. Distal socioeconomic determinants of child mortality operate through five main categories of proximate determinants: maternal factors (mother's age, parity, and birth spacing), environmental contaminants (routes of infection), nutrient deficiency, injury (unintentional and intentional), and personal illness control (preventive and curative health care). Mosley and Chen stress the importance of the synergistic effects of multiple determinants over time. Adapting this framework for the study of gender disparities, potential outcomes of son preference include differential maternal factors; differential injury, including female infanticide; differential exposure to infectious agents, which is least likely to be different for girls and boys in India; differential caloric, micronutrient, and macronutrient intake; and perhaps most importantly, differential access to preventive and curative health care. The combined effects of these disparities in the determinants of child mortality lead to excess female child mortality, which is most likely to manifest after the first year of life.

Moderating the pathway between son preference (lack of female entitlement) and its potential consequences are the contextual and individual characteristics that comprise Sen's capabilities. In Figure 3.1 these are shown at the bottom as resources to actualize son preference and include such factors as level of education, household wealth, mother's status in terms of autonomy and decision-making, and community development and services, including access to modern medical technology.

CHAPTER 4

RESEARCH METHODS

STUDY POPULATION

Two rounds of the Indian National Family Health Survey (NFHS), a Demographic and Health Survey (DHS) administered by the International Institute for Population Sciences (IIPS), have been completed. NFHS-1 was collected in 1992–1993 using the DHS II questionnaire and covering 89,777 ever-married women; NFHS-2 was collected in 1998–1999 using the DHS III questionnaire, interviewing 90,303 ever-married women.

The survey was implemented within each state and was designed to provide estimates for India as a whole, and at the state level, for rural and urban areas separately, as well as for regions within some of the larger states. A two-stage sample design was implemented in rural areas and a three-stage sample design in urban areas. For rural areas, in the first stage, villages served as the primary sampling units (PSUs) and were selected with probability proportional to population size. In the second stage of sampling, households within each PSU were systematically sampled with equal probability. In urban areas, census wards were selected with probability proportional to size at the first sampling stage, then within each sampled ward, one census enumeration block was randomly selected. In the third stage, households were systematically sampled with equal probability within each census block. All ever-married women aged 15–49 who were de facto residents of sampled households (i.e., women who stayed in the household the night before the survey) were interviewed, with an overall response rate of 96%.

Data from the birth history administered to women in both rounds of the NFHS was used to generate a dataset of births in the 15 years prior to interview, thus the dataset included births during the years 1977 to 1993 for NFHS-1 and the years 1983 to 1999 for NFHS-2. A preliminary analysis of these data show that there were 185,642 births reported in the 15-year period prior to the NFHS-1 interview and 177,004 births reported in the 15 years prior to the NFHS-2 interview. Of the 185,642 births reported in the 15 years prior to NFHS-1, 20,047 (10.8%) were reported to have died by 5 years of age. Similarly for NFHS-2, of the 177,004 births in the 15 years prior to interview, 17,155 (9.7%) were reported to have died by the age of 5.

DIFFERENTIAL RECALL OF FEMALE BIRTHS

When reporting a birth history, women tend to omit children who did not survive, especially children who died at an early age (United Nations, 1983). Because child mortality is higher for females than males in this setting, the result is a recall bias toward greater reporting of male births and lower reporting of female births. This bias is expected to intensify with the length of recall.

To determine the extent of differential recall of male births by length of recall, the 544,049 total births reported in both rounds of the NFHS were examined by calendar year of birth. NFHS-2 interviews occurred in 1998–1999, and NFHS-1 interviews in 1992–1993; thus, births that occurred in the same calendar year will differ by the length of recall in the two surveys. If the sex ratio at birth during the same calendar years differs as measured by the two surveys, this indicates a significant recall bias, and births of that recall length and longer should be excluded from the analysis. As shown in Table A.4.1, the sex ratio at birth did not differ by survey round until 1978–1982, which was prior to the broad availability of sex-determination tests. Births reported in NFHS-1 with a recall of 9–15 years have a sex ratio of 106.6, which is slightly higher than the expected biological value of 105–106, whereas births reported in NFHS-2 with a recall of 15–22 years have a sex ratio of 109.2 ($p = 0.06$). This recall length bias worsens for earlier calendar years: 1973–1977, with sex ratios of 106.1 and 113.2 for NFHS-1 and NFHS-2, respectively ($p < 0.001$). For calendar years prior to 1973, well before prenatal sex determination testing was available, both surveys demonstrate substantial recall bias with sex ratios of 111.9 and 113.3 ($p = 0.56$). As a result of this analysis, births reported to have occurred 15 years or more prior to interview were excluded from the analysis. Table A.4.2 shows the distribution of the 362,646 births in the 15 years prior to interview by survey round and calendar year. Of those 362,646 births,

344,740 births to usual residents of the surveyed households were included in the study.

Male Birth Proportion

Study Design

The first study objective is to examine correlates of and changes over time in sex-selective abortion, shown in the overall framework (Figure 3.1) as a prenatal consequence of son preference. Because a direct measure of sex-selective abortion is not available over a span of years and because the measure is subject to severe underreporting, a consequence of sex-selective abortion, namely the proportion of male births, was used as a proxy, as shown in Figure 4.1, where the circles represent latent, unmeasured variables, and the squares are manifest variables. A cross-sectional study design was used to identify characteristics associated with a higher proportion of male births during the period 1977–1999 and characteristics associated with a more rapid increase in male proportion of births over time. Births in the past 15 years reported on the birth histories in the two survey rounds were combined, comprising births over the interval from 1977–1999, and a cross-sectional analysis of the proportion of male births was performed.

Factors reported at the time of the survey may have changed, since the occurrence of the more distant births 10–15 years prior. Reverse causality is not likely, however, because the sex of the child, who if still living would be 10–15 years old, would not be likely to impact those factors, such as education of parents, household wealth, or female autonomy. It may be that later,

Figure 4.1. Analytical framework for testing the substitution hypothesis.

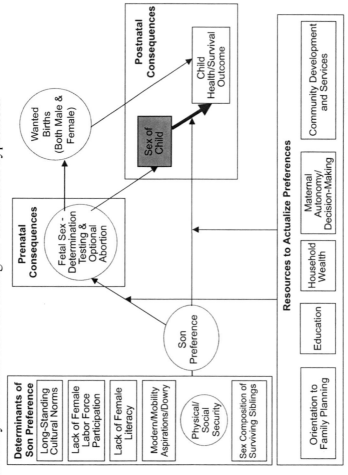

when those children are adults, their sex will have an impact on some of these factors; indeed, that is what the parents might expect and is itself a justification for son preference. By the age of 15, however, the expected benefits of sons are not likely to have manifested.

Hypotheses

The following characteristics, which are determinants of son preference, are hypothesized to be associated with a greater proportion of male births:

- Core Indo-Aryan cultural pattern
- Greater marital distance (spatial exogamy)
- Women's lack of labor force participation
- Higher birth orders
- Two or more surviving older sisters at the time of birth
- No surviving older brothers at the time of birth

Similarly, the following capability factors, which may affect the ability to realize son preferences, are hypothesized to be associated with a higher proportion of male births:

- Households where parents have more education
- Households with greater wealth (assets)
- Areas with greater access to medical technology

The hypothesis that there is expected to be a greater increase in male proportion of births over calendar time by the preceding list of determinants and capabilities was tested by a significant interaction term between the factor and calendar year of birth.

As found in prior studies, the hypothesis that the effect of women's labor force participation is greater in communities where the core Indo-Aryan cultural pattern prevails was tested with an interaction between women's labor force participation and cultural pattern. I hypothesized that there would be a greater increase in the male proportion of births over time in communities where women's labor force participation is low and the cultural pattern is core Indo-Aryan, which I tested with an interaction term between calendar year of birth, women's labor force participation, and cultural pattern. Mother's level of education and father's level of education were assessed in a similar fashion. Family size was not included as a control variable in this analysis because it would have confused the effects of differential stopping behavior and sex-selective abortion (Clark, 2000).

Derived Variables

Asset Index

To measure household wealth, an asset index was calculated based on ownership of agricultural land, livestock, consumer durables, and other household amenities reported on the household questionnaire. The index is identical to the standard of living index generally used in NFHS-1; because the same variables were also collected in NFHS-2, it was possible to calculate a consistent household index across both surveys. (The standard of living index commonly used in NFHS-2 includes a number of additional consumer goods, such as color television, telephone, and pieces of furniture, as well as household ownership).

Table A.4.4 displays the variables and codes from the two NFHS surveys used to construct a consistent asset index. Scores were assigned and summed as follows:

1. **House type:** 4 for pucca (high-quality materials such as bricks, tiles, cement, and concrete throughout, including roof, walls, and floor), 2 for semi-pucca (partly low-quality materials and partly high-quality materials), 0 for kachha (mud, thatch, or other low-quality materials).

2. **Toilet facility:** 4 for own flush toilet, 2 for public or shared flush toilet or own pit toilet, 1 for shared or public pit toilet, 0 for no facility.

3. **Source of lighting:** 2 for electricity, 1 for kerosene, gas, or oil, 0 for other source of lighting.

4. **Main fuel for cooking:** 2 for electricity, liquified natural gas, or biogas, 1 for coal, charcoal, or kerosene, 0 for other fuel.

5. **Source of drinking water:** 2 for pipe, hand pump, or well in residence/yard/plot, 1 for public tap, hand pump, or well, 0 for other water source.

6. **Separate room for cooking:** 1 for yes, 0 for no.

7. **Ownership of agricultural land:** 4 for 5 acres or more, 3 for 2.0–4.9 acres, 2 for less than 2 acres or acreage not known, 0 for no agricultural land.

8. **Ownership of irrigated land:** 2 if household owns at least some irrigated land, 0 for no irrigated land.

9. **Ownership of livestock:** 2 if household owns livestock, 0 for no livestock.

10. **Durable goods ownership:** 4 for a car or tractor, 3 each for a scooter/motorcycle or refrigerator, 2.5 for a television, 2 each for a bicycle, electric fan, radio/transistor, sewing machine, water pump, bullock cart, or thresher, 1 for a clock/watch.

Index scores ranged from 0–50.5 and were categorized by quintiles into low (0–7.5), lower middle (8.0–11.5), middle (12.0–15.5), higher middle (16.0–22.0), and high (22.5–50.5).

Number of Older Brothers and Sisters
Rather than utilizing the number of older siblings at the time of birth, a more specific variable was created to indicate the number of surviving older siblings at the approximate time of fetal sex determination, because this is the crucial time when a female fetus is at risk of being aborted. The time of fetal sex determination was estimated as 19 weeks prior to date of birth, which is approximately 20 weeks of gestation. Two variables—the number of surviving female siblings and the number of surviving male siblings—were computed.

Statistical Analysis
The data were first analyzed in a bivariate fashion to identify factors and covariates that are correlated with the response, which is the proportion of births that are male. The proportion of male births were computed and tabled by individual-level, family-level, and village-level characteristics. Bivariate associations were tested using the Pearson chi-squared statistic, corrected for the survey design using the second-order correction

of Rao and Scott (1984), and converted into an F-statistic using the *svytab* command in Stata version 8 software (Stata Corporation, 2003).

A multilevel logistic regression analysis was carried out to identify individual-level, family-level, and PSU-level characteristics independently associated with a higher proportion of male births during the period 1977–1999 and characteristics associated with a more rapid increase in male proportion of births over time. The *gllamm* module for Stata software was used for multilevel analyses (Rabe-Hesketh, Skrondal, & Pickles, 2002).

The first model run was a variance-components model (random-intercept model) to find the proportion of the variance attributable to family-level and PSU-level random effects:

$$\ln[p(\text{male})_{ijk} / (1-p(\text{male})_{ijk})] = \beta_{0jk}$$

where i indexes children, j indexes families, and k indexes PSUs. The second-level (family-level) equation is then defined as:

$$\beta_{0jk} = \beta_{0k} + \mu_{0jk}, \, \mu_{0jk} \sim N(0, \tau_{00})$$

And the third-level (PSU-level) equation is defined as:

$$\beta_{0k} = \gamma_{00} + \upsilon_{0k}, \, \upsilon_{0k} \sim N(0, \tau_{11})$$

The Wald test was used to determine the statistical significance of the variance of the random effects, τ_{00} and τ_{11}.

If significant family-level variability in male births were found (i.e., if τ_{00} is significantly different from zero) a logistic random intercept model with coefficient as outcome would be run, whereby family-level random effects (β_{0jk}) are regressed on the family-level covariates (Y_{jk}):

$$\text{logit}[p(\text{male})_{ijk}] = \beta_{0jk} + \beta_1 X_{ijk}$$

$$\beta_{0jk} = \beta_{0k} + \gamma_{01} Y_{jk} + \mu_{0jk}$$

Similarly, if there were significant PSU-level variability in male births (i.e., if τ_{00} is significantly different from zero), PSU-level random-effects (β_{0k}) would be regressed on PSU-level covariates (Z_k) to find the proportion of the PSU-level variance thus explained:

$$\beta_{0k} = \gamma_{00} + \gamma_{01} Z_k + \upsilon_{0k}$$

Model Building

Multivariate models were constructed using the method of purposeful selection of covariates. Variables significant at an alpha level of 0.25 in the bivariate analysis were initially included in the multivariate model, along with important control variables, including year of birth, geographic region, and socioeconomic status. Wald statistics were used to determine the statistical significance of each variable in the multivariate model. The variables that were no longer statistically significant in the presence of other covariates were removed (except for those variables identified as important control variables). A likelihood ratio test would usually be used to compare the reduced model to the initial model to assess the statistical significance of the removed covariates, but in this analysis, the likelihood ratio test cannot be used because the data are clustered (Skinner, 1989). In the next step, the variables originally omitted from the model because they were not statistically significant in the bivariate analysis were added to the regression model, one at a time, to assess statistical significance in the presence of the other covariates. Those with significant Wald statistics remained in the model. Interaction terms were constructed as specified by the research hypotheses and added to the model one at a time. Significant interaction terms as assessed by the Wald statistic remained in the model. Collinearity between covariates was assessed by a change of greater than 10% in the beta coefficient when the correlated variable was added to the model and by a substantial increase in the standard error of the beta coefficient.

Continuous variables, including birth year, household standard of living (asset index), distance to nearest hospital, distance to nearest town, and number of households in village were categorized by quintiles.

Eꜰꜰᴇᴄᴛ ᴏꜰ Sᴇx Sᴇʟᴇᴄᴛɪᴏɴ ᴏɴ Mᴏʀᴛᴀʟɪᴛʏ

Study Design
The second study objective is to investigate changes over time in gender differentials in child mortality and to determine if prenatal sex selection is having an effect on those differentials. As shown in Figure 4.1, an imbalance in the sex ratio of births is not the only consequence of prenatal sex selection but also affected is the wantedness of births—both male and female—which has been shown to affect child morbidity and mortality. Those girls born into families which practice prenatal sex

selection are more likely to be wanted than girls born into families which do not practice prenatal selection; their parents had the option of aborting the pregnancy but chose not to.

The contrast of interest in this study is the difference between male and female child mortality (bold line in Figure 4.1). Since the early 1980s in India, China, and South Korea, sex at birth is no longer a random process with a defined probability but is subject to selective forces. If those selective factors also influence postnatal outcomes, then they confound the relationship between sex of the baby and the outcomes. Conditioning on the selective factors is required to obtain an unbiased estimate of the effect of the child's sex on health and survival outcomes.

Rosenbaum and Rubin (1983) proposed a balancing score for studies where the *treatment* (in this case the sex of child) is not randomly assigned. In randomized experiments the response may be directly compared between two treatment groups because the individuals in each group are likely to be similar. In observational studies, the individuals exposed to one treatment are likely to differ systematically from those exposed to the other treatment; thus, a direct comparison of responses would be biased. A balancing score can be used to group individuals with similar characteristics from each treatment group so that meaningful comparisons can be made. The propensity score is the coarsest function of the observed pretreatment covariates that is a balancing score, and it is defined as the conditional probability of assignment to a particular treatment given a vector of observed covariates.

Using the results from the logistic regression analysis of male birth proportion, a propensity score was estimated for each birth as the posterior predictive probability of assignment to (or selection of) male gender for an individual with a vector of observed covariates. In other words, the propensity score tells us how likely it is that this particular birth is a boy, given a set of background factors that may predispose toward prenatal selection of a son. For example, a third birth to a well-educated urban family in 1995 has a higher probability of being a prenatally selected boy compared to a similar birth in 1980. The estimated propensity score reflects the vector of factors at multiple levels of measurement, which are correlated with prenatal sex selection and also with the subsequent wantedness of births. For example, a girl born as the third birth to a well-educated urban family in 1995 is more likely to be wanted than a girl born with the same background in 1980, because the parents were more likely to have had the option of sex-selective abortion and were predisposed to exercise that option. The propensity score was categorized into quintiles, which is based on Cochran's assessment that subclassification into five categories is sufficient to remove at least 90% of the bias when adjusting for a continuously distributed variable (Cochran, 1968).

Adjustment for the propensity score not only provides an unbiased estimate of gender differentials in mortality in settings where sex may be selected prenatally, it also allows for comparison of gender differentials in mortality between children born to parents who are more and less likely to opt for sex selection and allows for comparisons over time, as prenatal sex-selection has diffused.

Hypotheses

Change in the gender differential in child mortality over time was assessed by the statistical significance of a two-way interaction between gender and calendar year. A statistically significant and negatively signed interaction term between gender (1 = Female, 0 = Male) and calendar year would indicate a significant decline in the gender differential in child mortality over calendar time.

Gender differentials in child mortality were graphed by the quintile of the propensity score (from low propensity for sex-selective abortion to high propensity for sex-selective abortion) and by calendar year of birth, from 1977–1983 (before ultrasound technology was widely available) to 1999, the last year for which birth data is available.

The substitution hypothesis was tested by a three-way interaction term between year of birth, gender, and propensity score. If the interaction term were statistically significant and negatively signed, that would provide evidence that prenatal selection is substituting for postnatal mortality. As access to sex-selection technology diffuses over time, if substitution is occurring, then those with the highest propensity for sex-selection should experience disproportionately lower gender differentials, and that effect should intensify over time.

Because the psychological cost of prenatal discrimination is likely to be less than the psychological cost of postnatal discrimination, there may be families who would opt for the former but never the latter. For these families, sex-selective abortion *would not* have an impact upon gender differentials in child health and survival. In other words, the substitution hypothesis would not hold for these families. In families for whom postnatal discrimination is not too costly psychologically, or for whom the psychological costs are outweighed by other factors such as economic costs, sex-selective abortion *would* have an impact upon gender differentials in child health and survival; that is, they would substitute prenatal selection for postnatal excess female mortality. Three-way interactions between gender, propensity score, and family-level characteristics were assessed to identify factors that may predispose toward substitution.

For the purpose of policy recommendations and to understand the ages at which the greatest impact of prenatal sex-selection may occur, it is important to obtain estimates for each age segment, specifically, neonatal, postneonatal, and young child (ages 1–4). It is expected that the greatest effects of prenatal sex-selection on gender differentials in mortality will occur among young children, because that is the stage when social and behavioral mortality determinants predominate (Waldron, 1987).

Statistical Analysis

Separate logistic regression models were fitted for neonatal, postneonatal, and early child (age 1–4) mortality for births in the past 15 years reported in the NFHS-1 and NFHS-2 birth histories. Only those who survived the neonatal period were analyzed in the postneonatal model, and only those who survived the infant period were included in the young child model. The outcome variable is: $(0 = \text{survived}, 1 = \text{died})$.

The logistic model is specified as follows:

$$\ln[p(\text{died})_{ijk} / (1-p(\text{died})_{ijk})] = \beta_{0jk} + X\beta$$

where i indexes children, j indexes families, and k indexes PSUs. The second-level (family-level) equation is then defined as:

$$\beta_{0jk} = \beta_{0k} + \mu_{0jk}, \ \mu_{0jk} \sim N(0, \tau_{00})$$

And the third-level (PSU-level) equation is defined as:

$$\beta_{0k} = \gamma_{00} + \upsilon_{0k}, \upsilon_{0k} \sim N(0, \tau_{11})$$

The Wald test was used to determine the statistical significance of the variance of the random effects, τ_{00} and τ_{11}.

$X\beta$ = covariates and parameters as follows:

$$= \beta_0 + \beta_1 \text{Gender}_{ijk} + \beta_2 P1_{ijk} + \beta_3 P3_{ijk} + \beta_4 P4_{ijk} + \beta_5 P5_{ijk}$$
$$+ \beta_6 Y1_{ijk} + \beta_7 Y2_{ijk} + \beta_8 Y3_{ijk} + \beta_{X1} X_{1ijk} + \cdots + \beta_{XN} X_{Nijk}$$
$$+ \beta_{Z1} Z_{1ijk} + \cdots + \beta_{ZM} Z_{Mijk}$$

Gender (1 = female, 0 = male); P1 to P5 are dummy variables for quintiles of the propensity score, with P2 omitted as the referent category; Y1 to Y3 are dummy variables for calendar year of birth grouped 1977–1983, 1984–1989, 1990–1999; X_1 to X_N are N other covariates; Z_1 to Z_M are M interaction terms between gender and propensity score dummy variables, and between gender and calendar year dummy variables, and between gender, propensity score dummy variables and covariates; β_0 = the intercept; β_1 = regression coefficient for gender; k is the index for villages/census blocks, j is the index for families, and i is the index for individuals within groups.

Other covariates included in the model, which have been shown to be related to child survival, include preceding birth interval, mother's age, parity, as well parents' educational levels, and socioeconomic status.

The multilevel model was estimated with MLwiN 2.0 software using iterative generalized least squares (IGLS) with a quasi-likelihood estimation procedure and first-order marginal quasi-likelihood (MQL). The MQL method tends to bias estimates downward, but the model is more likely to converge, so the MQL method was first used, followed by the PQL method, using the MQL estimates as a starting point for the PQL interation. If the model was not able to converge using the PQL method, the final MQL estimates were used (Goldstein, 2003).

Study Design

In order to further elucidate the results of the mortality analyses, the proximate determinants of child mortality were analyzed to identify the processes and pathways through which prenatal sex selection may be exerting the greatest impact on infant and child mortality. Data on proximate determinants are available only for children born in the 3 years prior to interview who were still surviving at the time of the interview.

A cross-sectional study design was used to examine the difference between male and female outcomes. The outcomes of interest are full immunization by the age of 12 months, which measures preventive care; treatment for diarrhea or acute respiratory infection; which represents curative care; and a measure of compound morbidity, which combines nutrition and infection. Stunting is a measure of long-term nutritional deficiency, whereas wasting measures acute nutritional deficits or illness. Because it is the compounding of nutritional deficiency and infectious diseases which often lead to child deaths, an outcome of stunting or wasting combined with diarrhea or acute respiratory infection was analyzed. To summarize, three outcomes were analyzed: full immunization, treatment for either diarrhea or acute respiratory infection, and compound nutrition/infection morbidity.

Hypotheses

Change in the gender differential in each of the outcome measures over time was assessed by the statistical significance of a two-way interaction term between gender and calendar year. A two-way interaction term between gender and propensity score was used to assess the impact of prenatal selection on gender differentials in the outcome measure of interest. If the interaction term were statistically significant and negatively signed, it provided evidence that prenatal sex selection is effecting a decrease in gender differentials in the outcome of interest.

Statistical Analysis

Logistic regression analysis was used to analyze the binary outcomes of lack of full immunization, untreated illness, and presence of nutrition/infection compound morbidity, as described in detail in the section on statistical analysis of mortality outcomes.

SAMPLE SIZE CONSIDERATIONS

Male Birth Proportion

To detect a 5% difference between two groups in the proportion of births that are male would require a sample size of 5,864 in each group, assuming a two-sided significance level (alpha) of 0.05, 80% power, and a proportion in one of the groups that is equal to 0.514. This sample size calculation for a difference between two proportions uses a normal approximation to the binomial distribution with a continuity correction. The 5% minimum difference detectable in proportions would correspond to a difference between a sex ratio at birth of 1.055 and 1.172.

Because this is a complex survey design, the sample size needs to be adjusted for the design effect. Design effects for various survey measures are published, however, not for the outcome of sex of births. The number of children ever born had the following values for design effect: urban 2.445, rural 1.741, total 1.947, and number of children surviving: urban 2.371, rural 1.606, total 1.806 (International Institute for Population Sciences and ORC Macro, 2000). Thus, assuming a maximum design effect of 2.5, the required sample size in each group increased to 14,660. The number of births included in this study is 362,646; 73% of births occurred in rural areas, so there will be adequate statistical power to perform subgroups analyses over time in rural areas (see Table 4.1).

Table 4.1. Number of births and deaths by urban/rural residence and calendar year.

Year of Birth	Births	Deaths		
		Neonatal	Postneonatal	Young Child
Urban:				
1977–1982	16,587	665	430	322
1983–1987	30,367	1,136	732	567
1988–1993	36,266	1,201	634	421
1994–1999	15,384	459	222	117
Total Urban	98,604	3,461	2,018	1,427
Rural:				
1977–1982	40,839	2,403	1,709	1,649
1983–1987	77,924	4,415	2,826	2,667
1988–1993	100,771	4,967	2,845	2,394
1994–1999	44,508	1,959	1,070	676
Total Rural	264,042	13,744	8,450	7,386

In urban areas there will be adequate statistical power to detect a 10% increase in the proportion of male births over time, analyzing by subgroups, which should be sufficient because the effect size is hypothesized to be much larger in urban areas where there is greater access to technology for sex-selective abortion. To detect a 10% difference between two groups in the proportion of births that are male would require a sample size of 1,887 in each group, assuming a two-sided significance level (a) of 0.05, 80% power, and a proportion in one of the groups that is equal to 0.514. Adjusting for the estimated design effect of 2.5 would result in a sample size of 4,718 in each group. The 10% minimum difference detectable would correspond to a difference between a sex ratio at birth of 1.055 and 1.301.

Effect of Sex Selection on Mortality

Neonatal Mortality

The hypothesized effect size may be specified based on the ratio of the female-to-male probability of neonatal death, which in urban areas is 0.76 and in rural areas is 0.90 (IIPS and ORC Macro, 2000). The sample size available is adequate to detect a 30% difference in survival (effect size of 1.3) in urban areas which would require 7128 subjects in each group, adjusted for the design effect of 2.5, with 80% power and a two-sided alpha of 0.05. In rural areas, the minimum detectable difference in survival is 20%.

Postneonatal Mortality

In urban areas the ratio of female-to-male probability of post-neonatal death is 0.97, and in rural areas the ratio is 1.13 (IIPS and ORC Macro, 2000). Given the number of subjects available, there will be adequate power to detect a minimum effect size of 1.4 in urban areas, with 80% power and a two-sided alpha of 0.05 and with a minimum effect size of 1.2 in rural areas.

Young Child Mortality

In urban areas the ratio of female-to-male probability of young child (1–4) mortality is 1.35, and in rural areas the ratio is 1.50 (IIPS and ORC Macro, 2000). Given the number of subjects available, there will be adequate power to detect a minimum effect size of 1.4 in urban areas, with 80% power and a two-sided alpha of 0.05 and with a minimum effect size of 1.2 in rural areas.

EFFECT OF SEX SELECTION ON HEALTH CARE AND MORBIDITY

Preliminary analysis of the survey data show prevalence of the outcomes to be as follows: Sixty percent were not fully vaccinated, of 20% with diarrhea or acute respiratory infection, 40% received no medical treatment, and 15% were suffering from compound nutrition/infection morbidity based on 34,122 children born 1989–1993 and 30,984 children born 1995–1999. With 80% power and a two-sided alpha of 0.05, adjusted for the design effect of 2.5, the study will be able to detect a minimum difference of 10% for the outcome of not fully vaccinated, a minimum difference of 50% in lack of curative treatment for diarrhea or acute respiratory infection, and a minimum difference of 30% in compound morbidity.

CHAPTER 5

CHARACTERISTICS ASSOCIATED WITH MALE BIRTH PROPORTION

The objective of this study was to identify correlates of sex-selective abortion in India, to investigate changes over calendar time in levels of sex-selective abortion, and to determine if correlates have changed over time. Because a direct measure of sex-selective abortion is not available, the proportion of male births will serve as a proxy measure. Where sex-selective abortion is more frequent, the proportion of male births will be elevated above the natural proportion of 0.513, and the sex ratio will be elevated above 1.05.

The birth history administered to women in both rounds of the NFHS was used to generate a dataset of births in the 15 years prior to interview to women who are usual household residents.

The dataset thus includes births during the years 1977 to 1993 for NFHS-1 and 1983 to 1999 for NFHS-2. There were 176,478 births to usual residents reported in the 15-year period prior to the NFHS-1 interview and 168,262 births to usual residents reported in the 15 years prior to the NFHS-2 interview, resulting in a total of 344,740 births to 131,122 mothers residing in 120,255 households within 6,688 primary sampling units (PSUs) consisting of villages or urban census blocks. The majority (73%) of births occurred in rural areas: 250,745 births to 91,306 mothers in 4,262 PSUs.

SAMPLE CHARACTERISTICS AND BIVARIATE ASSOCIATIONS WITH MALE BIRTH

Child-Level Factors

Frequency distributions of child-level characteristics and bivariate association with male birth are shown in Table 5.1. Birth year ranged from 1977–1999 and was categorized into quintiles: 1977–1983, 1984–1986, 1987–1989, 1990–1992, and 1993–1999. Nearly one quarter of births were preceded by a birth interval of less than 2 years, 26% had a birth interval of 24–35 months, and 24% were born after an interval of 3 years or more. Twenty-six percent were first births, 23% were second born, 18% were third born, and 33% were fourth or higher birth order. Nearly half of the children (49.4%) had no surviving older brothers at the time when they were at approximately 20 weeks of gestation, one third (31%) had one older brother, and 20% had two or more surviving older brothers. Similarly, 49% had no surviving older sisters, 29% had only one older sister, and 23% had two or more older sisters surviving. The highest proportion of children (36%) were born to mothers aged 20–24 years, whereas 25% were born

Table 5.1. Child-level variables: Frequency distribution and male birth proportion.

Characteristic	Number of Births	Percent of Total (Weighted)	Proportion Male (Weighted)	p-value
Year of Birth (Quintiles):				
1977–1983	61,706	20.0%	0.517	
1984–1986	63,808	20.5%	0.515	
1987–1989	64,173	20.2%	0.521	
1990–1992	63,960	19.9%	0.513	
1993–1999	64,849	19.4%	0.518	0.16
Length of Preceding Birth Interval:				
N/A (First Birth)	82,640	25.6%	0.516	
<24 Months	74,051	24.2%	0.518	
24–35 Months	84,542	26.4%	0.517	
36+ Months	77,260	23.8%	0.517	0.95
Length of Subsequent Birth Interval:				
<24 Months	63,923	21.9%	0.489	
24–35 Months	71,152	22.4%	0.496	
36+ months	57,164	17.8%	0.510	
N/A (Last Birth)	126,255	37.9%	0.549	<0.001

(continued)

Table 5.1. Child-level variables: Frequency distribution and male birth proportion. *(continued)*

Characteristic	Number of Births	Percent of Total (Weighted)	Proportion Male (Weighted)	p-value
Birth Order:				
1	82,356	25.5%	0.516	
2	76,130	23.3%	0.519	
3	58,748	18.1%	0.518	
4+	101,262	33.1%	0.516	0.78
Number of Older Brothers Born:				
None	144,028	44.4%	0.518	
One	95,998	29.8%	0.518	
Two or More	78,470	25.8%	0.513	0.09
Number of Older Sisters Born:				
None	143,647	44.5%	0.516	
One	88,482	27.6%	0.517	
Two or More	86,367	27.9%	0.519	0.59

Surviving Older Brothers:				
None	157,397	49.4%	0.519	
One	99,164	30.9%	0.518	
Two or More	61,935	19.8%	0.512	0.04
Surviving Older Sisters:				
None	155,046	48.8%	0.516	
One	91,186	28.6%	0.517	
Two or More	72,264	22.7%	0.520	0.23
Mother's Age at Time of Birth:				
<20	73,936	26.2%	0.517	
20–24	117,936	36.2%	0.516	
25–29	77,171	22.7%	0.518	
30–34	35,776	10.7%	0.519	
35+	13,677	4.2%	0.515	0.95

to teenage mothers, 23% to mothers in their late twenties, and 15% to mothers 30 years and older.

Bivariate associations of child-level characteristics with the proportion of male births were assessed for statistical significance. The length of the subsequent birth interval was significantly associated with male birth proportion. Only 0.489 of the births followed by a shorter interval (<24 months) were male, compared to 0.510 of the births followed by a longer interval of 36 months or more, and the highest proportion of male births (0.549) was found among final births, which is a reflection of differential stopping behavior rather than sex-selective abortion (p < 0.001). There was also a statistically significant association (p = 0.04) between the proportion of male births and the number of surviving older brothers at the time of earliest fetal sex determination by ultrasound (approximately 20 weeks of gestation). Among births with no surviving older brothers, 0.519 were male; among those with only one surviving older brother 0.518 were male, compared to 0.512 of births with two or more surviving older brothers.

Family-Level Factors

Table 5.2 displays frequency distributions of the family-level variables and the proportion of male births in each category. Eighty-one percent of families were Hindu, 13% were Muslim, 2.4% were Christian, and all other religions combined accounted for 3.4% of families. Sixteen percent of families belonged to scheduled castes, 9% belonged to scheduled tribes, and 75% belonged to neither.

The majority of mothers (62%) were illiterate, 18% had some primary schooling, 7% completed middle school, and only 12%

Table 5.2. Family-level variables: Frequency distribution and male birth proportion.

Characteristic	Number of Families	Percent of Total	Number of Births	Proportion Male (Weighted)	p-value
Religion:					
Hindu	100,938	81.2%	260,675	0.518	
Muslim	15,355	13.0%	46,800	0.508	
Christian	8,362	2.4%	21,280	0.516	
Other	6,401	3.4%	15,819	0.532	<0.001
Scheduled Caste/Tribe:					
Scheduled Caste	19,168	15.7%	53,500	0.519	
Scheduled Tribe	16,839	9.2%	47,836	0.513	
Neither	94,633	75.1%	241,888	0.517	0.28
Household Standard of Living (Quintiles):					
Low	21,975	19.6%	63,623	0.517	
Lower Middle	24,500	20.1%	70,674	0.515	
Middle	24,630	19.2%	68,714	0.512	
Higher Middle	27,884	20.2%	71,384	0.517	
High	32,133	20.8%	70,345	0.524	0.01

(continued)

Table 5.2. Family-level variables: Frequency distribution and male birth proportion. *(continued)*

Characteristic	Number of Families	Percent of Total	Number of Births	Proportion Male (Weighed)	p-value
Mother's Education:					
Illiterate	75,332	62.4%	219,927	0.515	
< Middle School	25,434	18.2%	63,865	0.519	
Middle School	11,173	7.4%	24,613	0.528	
High School+	19,169	12.1%	36,298	0.523	0.002
Father's Education:					
Illiterate	39,036	32.8%	115,658	0.517	
< Middle School	34,664	27.1%	94,250	0.513	
Middle School	17,884	12.6%	45,225	0.517	
High School+	39,060	27.5%	88,211	0.522	0.02
Mother's Labor Force Participation:					
None	83,597	63.0%	215,633	0.518	
Noncash	17,677	12.5%	50,486	0.516	
Cash	29,796	24.5%	78,471	0.514	0.17

Mother's Residence Here

Before/After Marriage:

Lived Here Before Marriage	50,105	37.2%	130,379	0.518
Moved Here at Marriage	44,688	36.1%	117,356	0.514
Moved Here After Marriage	36,329	26.8%	97,005	0.520
				0.04

Mother Tongue:

Group 1	74,024	59.6%	204,533	0.519
Group 2	8,006	7.7%	18,190	0.518
Group 4	20,853	20.9%	46,410	0.512
Other	28,224	11.9%	75,558	0.513
				0.02

completed high school. Fathers were somewhat better educated, with 28% completing high school, 13% completing middle school, and 27% with some primary schooling, yet a full third of fathers remained illiterate. The majority of mothers (63%) did not participate in the labor force, whereas 24% worked for cash, and 12% worked in the labor force but did not receive wages.

As a measure of patrilocal exogamy, the time elapsed since moving to current locality was compared to the number of years of marriage. Thirty-seven percent of mothers resided in their present locality prior to marriage and therefore, did not practice patrilocal exogamy. A similar proportion (36%) moved there at the time of their marriage and therefore, were likely to have practiced patrilocal exogamy. Another 27% of the mothers reported moving to the present locality at some point after their marriage; thus, it was not possible to determine whether these women had practiced patrilocal exogamy.

The native language, or mother tongue, was grouped according to cultural Indo-Aryan core/Dravidian status (Agnihotri, 1999). Group 1 includes Hindi, Bengali, Punjabi, Gujarati, Urdu, and Kashmiri and represents the core Aryan cultural pattern. Group 2 includes Marathi, Oriya, and Konkani and represents the Southern Indo-Aryan cultural pattern. Group 4 includes the Southern languages of Telegu, Tamil, Kannada, and Malayalam and represents the Dravidian cultural pattern. The residual category includes Assamese, Sindhi, English, and all other native tongues not falling into the first three groups. The majority of families (60%) were native speakers of languages falling into Group 1, and another 8% of families had mother tongues falling into Group 2. Group 4 languages were spoken by 21% of families, and 12% fell into the "other" category.

The family-level characteristics found to be significantly associated with the proportion of male births included: religion, household standard of living, both mother's and father's level of education, mother's residence before/after marriage, and mother tongue. Hindus (0.518) and Christians (0.516) had a higher proportion of male births than did Muslims (0.508), but by far the highest proportion was found among those classified as "other" (0.532) ($p < 0.001$). Included in the "other" category were Sikhs, with an extremely high proportion of 0.538 births being male.

Those in the highest quintile of the standard of living index had a higher proportion of male births (0.524) compared to the four lower quintiles, with proportions ranging from 0.512–0.517 ($p = 0.01$). Mothers with a middle school (0.528) and a high school (0.523) education had higher levels of male births than illiterate women (0.515) or women who did not complete middle school (0.519) ($p = 0.002$). Similarly, fathers with a high school education had a higher proportion of male births (0.522) than men with less than a high school education (0. 513–0. 517) ($p = 0.02$).

Contrary to the hypothesized relationship, the lowest proportion of male births were found among women who were likely to have practiced patrilocal exogamy (0.514) compared to women who lived in the same location before marriage (0.518) and women who moved to their current location after marriage (0.520) ($p = 0.04$), perhaps reflecting an effect of mobility. As hypothesized, those speaking native languages falling into Groups 1 and 2 were found to have a higher proportion of male births: 0.519 and 0.518, respectively, whereas those speaking Group 4 and "other" languages had low rates of male births (0.512 and 0.513, respectively) ($p = 0.02$), reflecting cultural as well as regional influences.

PSU-Level Factors

PSU-level characteristics are shown in Table 5.3. Two-thirds of the PSUs were located in rural areas, and one-third were located in urban areas. The geographic regions used in the study are shown in Map 5.1. The Central region of the country (Madhya Pradesh, Uttar Pradesh, Bihar, and Rajasthan) comprised 29% of sampled PSUs, followed by the Northern region (Haryana, New Delhi, Himachal Pradesh, Jammu, and Punjab) with 18%, the Southern region (Andhra Pradesh, Karnataka, Kerala, and Tamil Nadu) with 17%, the Northeast (Assam, Arunachal Pradesh, Manipur, Meghalaya, Mizoram, Nagaland, Sikkim, and Tripura) with 14%, the Western region (Goa, Gujarat, and Maharashtra) with 13%, and the Eastern region (Orissa and West Bengal) with 9% of sampled PSUs.

The predominant mother tongue in each PSU was the language spoken by the majority of respondents. The majority of PSUs (55%) had a preponderance of Group 1 language speakers, whereas 22% of PSUs were dominated by speakers of "other" languages, 16% by Group 4 languages, and 7% of PSU were populated predominantly with those who spoke Group 2 languages.

In rural PSUs, village surveys were used to assess the accessibility to health facilities and other services. Among rural PSUs, 14% of villages had a primary health center, 16% had a mobile health unit, and 79% had a hospital within 21 kilometers. Seventy-nine percent of villages had a town within 25 kilometers, the majority of villages had electricity (83%), and 85% had at least one television within the village.

PSU-level characteristics found to be significantly associated with the proportion of births that were male included geographic region ($p < 0.001$) and proximity to a town ($p = 0.013$). The North

Map 5.1. Geographic regions of India.

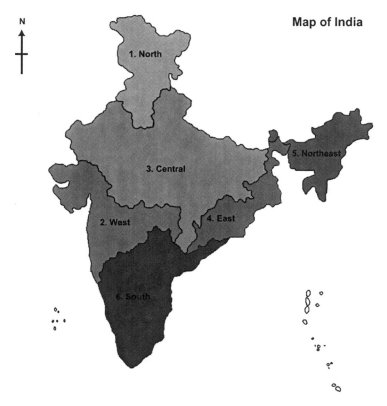

region had, by far, the highest proportion of male births (0.530), followed by the Central region (0.519), the Northeast (0.518), and the West (0.516). As expected, low male birth proportions were found in the South (0.512) and the East (0.510). Those villages located within 25 kilometers of a town were found to have a higher proportion of male births (0.516) compared to villages 25 kilometers or further from a town (0.511).

Table 5.3. PSU-level variables: Frequency distribution and male birth proportion.

Characteristic	Number of PSUs	Percent of Total	Number of Births	Proportion Male (Weighted)	p-value
Urban/Rural Residence:					
Urban	2,426	36.3%	93,995	0.520	0.12
Rural	4,262	63.7%	250,745	0.516	
Region:					
Region 1: North	1,217	18.2%	54,105	0.530	
Region 2: West	845	12.6%	35,690	0.516	
Region 3: Central	1,964	29.4%	129,773	0.519	
Region 4: East	599	9.0%	31,430	0.510	
Region 5: Northeast	927	13.9%	43,777	0.518	
Region 6: South	1,136	17.0%	49,965	0.512	<0.001
Predominant Mother Tongue:					
Group 1	3,680	55.0%	204,299	0.518	
Group 2	474	7.1%	18,575	0.518	
Group 4	1,087	16.3%	47,410	0.512	
Other	1,447	21.6%	74,456	0.517	0.15
Primary Health Center in Village:					
No	3,587	86.0%	211,233	0.515	
Yes	586	14.0%	32,289	0.520	0.15

Mobile Health Unit in Village:				
No	3,543	83.5%	203,814	0.516
Yes	698	16.5%	43,147	0.515	0.76
Nearest Hospital to Village (Quintiles):				
0–3 km	960	23.1%	54,057	0.515
4–7 km	829	20.0%	49,257	0.517
8–12 km	801	19.3%	48,438	0.517
13–21 km	734	17.7%	42,941	0.515
≥22 km	832	20.0%	49,606	0.517	0.94
Nearest Town to Village (Quintiles):				
0–5 km	926	22.0%	53,121	0.516
6–9 km	724	17.2%	43,879	0.520
10–14 km	790	18.8%	46,393	0.515
15–24 km	918	21.8%	52,448	0.519
≥25 km	855	20.3%	52,019	0.511	0.09
Electricity in Village:				
No	732	17.1%	46,270	0.518
Yes	3,544	82.9%	200,881	0.516	0.43

(continued)

Table 5.3. PSU-level variables: Frequency distribution and male birth proportion. *(continued)*

Characteristic	Number of PSUs	Percent of Total	Number of Births	Proportion Male (Weighted)	p-value
Television in Village:					
No	626	14.9%	36,177	0.513	
Yes	3,582	85.1%	206,804	0.516	0.33
Number of Households in Village (Quintiles):					
<125	932	22.2%	47,070	0.516	
125–248	820	19.5%	47,570	0.519	
249–400	837	20.0%	49,144	0.516	
401–744	740	17.6%	44,510	0.515	
745–8,930	866	20.6%	47,874	0.516	0.91

Note. Nearly all of the rural PSUs were comprised of one village. However, 75 PSUs were comprised of two villages, and one PSU included three villages; hence, the number of villages is slightly greater than the number of rural PSUs.

INDEPENDENT ASSOCIATIONS WITH MALE BIRTH

A random intercept logistic regression model was run to find the variance components at the family and PSU levels. The variance at the family level was estimated as 0.000002 with standard error 0.00008, and the variance at the PSU level was estimated as 0.000002 with standard error 0.0002. Thus, no significant random variability was found in probability of a male birth at the family or PSU levels, as reflected in Figure 5.1 and Figure 5.2, which show the empirical Bayes estimates of the probability of male birth versus the observed probability of male birth by family and PSU, respectively.

The coefficient estimates from a fixed effects logistic regression model with robust standard errors are shown in Table 5.4.

Figure 5.1. Estimated versus observed probability of male birth in family.

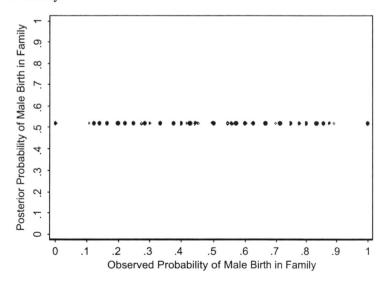

The individual-level factors found to be independently associated with male birth were: having no surviving older brothers compared to having two or more (p = 0.02), and a negative association with having no surviving older sisters compared to having two or more (p = 0.01). Year of birth was not independently associated with male birth, nor were the length of the preceding birth interval or mother's age at time of birth. The length of the subsequent birth interval was excluded from the model because it is a reflection of stopping behavior rather than sex-selective abortion.

Two family-level factors were found to be independently associated with male birth. Being born into a Muslim household was negatively associated with male birth compared to a Hindu

Figure 5.2. Estimated versus observed probability of male birth in PSU.

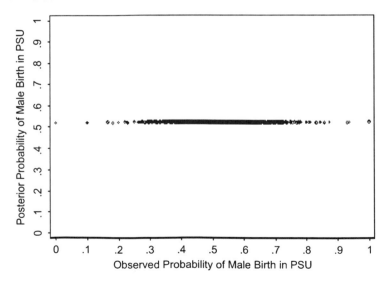

Table 5.4. Coefficient estimates from logistic regression model of male birth proportion, main effects only.

Characteristic	Coefficient (SE)	p-value
Individual Level		
Year of Birth (Quintiles):		
1977–1983	(Referent)	—
1984–1986	−0.0075 (0.0132)	0.57
1987–1989	0.0139 (0.0133)	0.30
1990–1992	−0.0191 (0.0132)	0.15
1993–1999	−0.0001 (0.0133)	0.99
Surviving Older Brothers:		
None	0.0271 (0.0112)	0.02
One	0.0213 (0.0120)	0.08
Two or More	(Referent)	
Surviving Older Sisters:		
None	−0.0280 (0.0109)	0.01
One	−0.0206 (0.0116)	0.08
Two or More	(Referent)	
Family Level		
Religion:		
Hindu	(Referent)	—
Muslim	−0.0402 (0.0118)	0.001
Christian	−0.0046 (0.0254)	0.86
Other	0.0312 (0.0220)	0.16
Mother's Education:		
Illiterate/< Middle School	(Referent)	—
Middle School	0.0485 (0.0172)	0.01
High School+	0.0232 (0.0140)	0.10
PSU Level		
Region:		
Region 1: North	0.0624 (0.0141)	<0.001
Region 2: West	0.0166 (0.0156)	0.29
Region 3: Central	0.0364 (0.0117)	0.002

(continued)

Table 5.4. Coefficient estimates from logistic regression model of male birth proportion, main effects only. *(continued)*

Characteristic	Coefficient (SE)	p-value
Region:		
Region 4: East	−0.0018 (0.0160)	0.91
Region 5: Northeast	0.0356 (0.0165)	0.03
Region 6: South	(Referent)	—
Nearest Town to Village:		
0–24 km	(Referent)	—
>25 km	−0.0301 (.0114)	0.01

household (p = 0.001), and mothers with a middle-school level of education were more likely to have sons compared to illiterate mothers (p = 0.005). Interestingly, mothers educated through at least high school were not significantly more likely to give birth to male children. The father's level of education was not independently associated with male birth. Scheduled caste or tribe status, the household standard of living, mother's labor force participation, and mobility were also not independently associated with a preponderance of male births.

PSU-level factors independently associated with male birth in this model were geographic regions located in the North (p < 0.001), Central (p = 0.002), or Northeast (p = 0.03) compared to the South and location in a city, a town, or a village within 25 kilometers of town compared to locations 25 kilometers or further from a town (p = 0.008). The predominant mother tongue spoken in a PSU was not independently associated with male birth, neither were the presences of a primary health center, a mobile clinic, a hospital in the village, nor the presence of either electric service or televisions. To assess changes over time in the effect of covariates that were significantly associated with male birth proportion, interaction terms were entered into the model. As shown in Table 5.5, significant effect changes over time were found for the number of surviving older brothers, the number of surviving older sisters, and the mother's level of education. Adjusted odds ratios (AOR) and 95% confidence intervals (CI) for the main effects in the model are shown in Figure 5.3. Relative to Hindus, Muslims were less likely to have male births (AOR 0.96, 95% CI 0.94–0.98). Births in the North (AOR 1.06, 95% CI 1.04–1.09), in the Central (AOR 1.04, 95% CI 1.01–1.06), and Northeast (AOR 1.04, 95% CI 1.00–1.07) regions were more likely to be male, and births occurring in villages 25 kilometers or more from a town were less likely to be male (AOR 0.97, 95% CI 0.95–0.99).

The significant interactions with year of birth from the logistic regression model are displayed in Figures 5.4–5.9, which show how the adjusted odds ratios changed over calendar time. Figure 5.4 shows that male birth did not become more likely among those with no surviving older brothers until the 1990s. In the period from 1990–1992, male birth was 5% more likely for those with no surviving older brothers compared to those with two or more surviving older brothers (AOR = 1.05, 95% CI 1.00–1.11), and in 1993–1999 male birth was 9% more likely (AOR = 1.09, 95% CI 1.04–1.15). As Figure 5.5 shows, there was little change over time in the odds ratio for those with only one surviving older brother compared to those with two or more older brothers, and the odds ratio was not significantly elevated during any of the time periods.

Table 5.5. Coefficient estimates from logistic regression model of male birth proportion, with interaction terms.

Characteristic	Coefficient (SE)	p-value
Individual-Level		
Year of Birth (Quintiles):		
1977–1983	(Referent)	—
1984–1986	0.0258 (0.0367)	0.48
1987–1989	0.0954 (0.0364)	0.01
1990–1992	0.0140 (0.0368)	0.70
1993–1999	0.0107 (0.0363)	0.77
Surviving Older Brothers:		
None	0.0109 (0.0255)	0.67
One	0.0326 (0.0274)	0.23
Two or More	(Referent)	—
Surviving Older Sisters:		
None	0.0327 (0.0253)	0.20
One	0.0164 (0.0273)	0.55
Two or More	(Referent)	—
Family-Level		
Religion:		
Hindu	(Referent)	—
Muslim	−0.0402 (0.0118)	0.001
Christian	−0.0034(0.0255)	0.89
Other	0.0317 (0.0221)	0.15
Mother's Education:		
< Middle School	(Referent)	—
Middle School	0.057 (0.0407)	0.16
High School+	−0.0316(0.0348)	0.36
PSU-Level		
Region:		
Region 1: North	0.0624 (0.0142)	<0.001
Region 2: West	0.0168 (0.0156)	0.28
Region 3: Central	0.0370 (0.0117)	0.002

(continued)

Table 5.5. Coefficient estimates from logistic regression model of male birth proportion, with interaction terms. *(continued)*

Characteristic	Coefficient (SE)	p-value
Region:		
Region 4: East	−0.0013 (0.0161)	0.93
Region 5: Northeast	0.0358 (0.0165)	0.03
Region 6: South	(Referent)	—
Nearest Town to Village:		
0–24 km	(Referent)	—
>25 km	−0.0313 (0.0114)	0.006
Interactions		
Surviving Older Brothers*		
Year of Birth:		
None * 1984–1986	−0.0220 (0.0356)	0.54
None * 1987–1989	−0.0098 (0.0357)	0.79
None * 1990–1992	0.0415 (0.0366)	0.26
None * 1993–1999	0.0769 (0.0362)	0.03
One * 1984–1986	−0.0256 (0.0383)	0.50
One * 1987–1989	−0.0117 (0.0374)	0.75
One * 1990–1992	−0.0073 (0.0390)	0.85
One * 1993–1999	−0.0053 (0.0378)	0.89
Surviving Older Sisters*		
Year of Birth:		
None * 1984–1986	−0.0343 (0.0349)	0.33
None * 1987–1989	−0.1103 (0.0350)	0.002
None * 1990–1992	−0.0644 (0.0354)	0.07
None * 1993–1999	−0.0969 (0.0351)	0.006
One * 1984–1986	−0.0021 (0.0378)	0.95
One * 1987–1989	−0.0695 (0.0384)	0.07
One * 1990–1992	−0.0702 (0.0371)	0.06
One * 1993–1999	−0.0453 (0.0375)	0.23
Mother's Education*		
Year of Birth:		
Middle School * 1984–1986	0.0282 (0.0566)	0.62
Middle School * 1987–1989	−0.0239 (0.0550)	0.66

(continued)

Table 5.5. Coefficient estimates from logistic regression model of male birth proportion, with interaction terms. *(continued)*

Characteristic	Coefficient (SE)	p-value
Mother's Education*		
Year of Birth:		
Middle School * 1990–1992	–0.0366 (0.0544)	0.50
Middle School * 1993–1999	–0.0054 (0.0530)	0.92
High School+ * 1984–1986	0.0211 (0.0484)	0.66
High School+ * 1987–1989	0.0394 (0.0479)	0.41
High School+ * 1990–1992	0.0432 (0.0469)	0.36
High School+ * 1993–1999	0.1323 (0.0451)	0.003

Note. Hosmer-Lemeshow goodness-of-fit test = 14.06 (8df), p = 0.08.

Change over time in the odds of male birth for those with no surviving older sisters compared to those with two or more surviving older sisters is displayed in Figure 5.6. The adjusted odds ratio did not fall below the null value of 1.00 until the late 1980s. Male births in families with no surviving older sisters were 8% less likely in 1987–1989 (AOR 0.92, 95% CI 0.88–0.97), 3% less likely in 1990–1992 (AOR 0.97, 95% CI 0.92–1.02), and 6% less likely in 1993–1999 (AOR 0.94, 95% CI 0.89–0.98). A similar trend in the odds of male birth was observed for those families with only one surviving older sister, with significantly reduced odds ratios for 1987–1989 (AOR 0.95, 95% CI 0.90–0.99), 1990–1992 (AOR 0.95, 95% CI 0.90–0.99), and an insignificantly lower adjusted odds ratio in 1993–1999 (AOR 0.97, 95% CI 0.92–1.02).

The effect of mother's level of education on the probability of male birth changed over time. Births to mothers with a middle school education compared to illiterate mothers had adjusted odds ratios 2% to 9% above 1.00 for each time period, although they were statistically significant only for the 1984

Figure 5.3. Adjusted odds ratios (95% CI) for main effects independently associated with the proportion of male births.

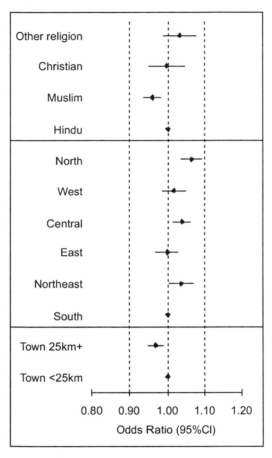

to 1986 time period. The adjusted odds ratio point estimate increased slightly over time for mothers with a high school education, from 0.97 in 1977–1983, 0.99 in 1984–1986, and 1.01 in 1987–1989 and 1990–1992. Then in 1993–1999 it jumped to 1.11 (95% CI 1.05–1.17).

Figure 5.4. Change over time in the adjusted odds ratio of male birth for those with no surviving older brothers versus those with two or more surviving older brothers.

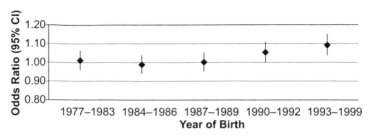

Figure 5.5. Change over time in the adjusted odds ratio of male birth for those with only one surviving older brother versus those with two or more surviving older brothers.

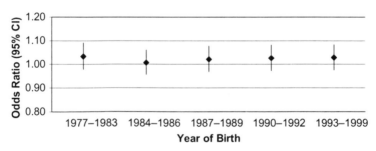

Figure 5.6. Change over time in the adjusted odds ratio of male birth for those with no surviving older sisters versus those with two or more surviving older sisters.

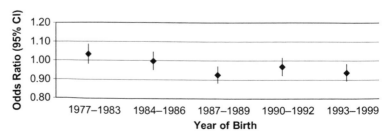

Figure 5.7. Change over time in the adjusted odds ratio of male birth for those with only one surviving older sister versus those with two or more surviving older sisters.

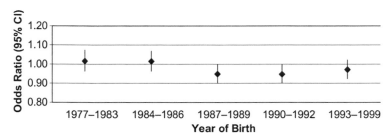

Figure 5.8. Change over time in the adjusted odds ratio of male birth for those with a middle school educated mother versus those with an illiterate mother.

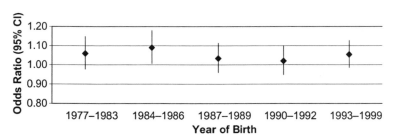

Figure 5.9. Change over time in the adjusted odds ratio of male birth for those with a high school educated mother versus those with an illiterate mother.

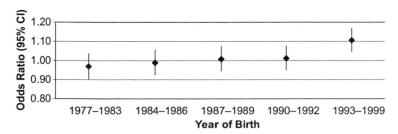

DISCUSSION

As hypothesized, several of the determinants of son preference were found to be associated with a greater proportion of male births in this study. Core Indo-Aryan cultural pattern was represented by three variables: geographic region, mother tongue, and religion. Male births were significantly more likely in the North, Central, and Northeast regions. Parents with native tongues falling into Group 1 (Indo-Aryan core and Central Rajasthani) and Group 2 (Southern Indo-Aryan) had a higher prevalence of male births, and native speakers of Group 4 (Dravidian) had a lower prevalence of male births. Because this variable is highly correlated with state of residence (Group 1 and Group 2 languages are predominantly spoken in the North and Central regions), it was no longer statistically significant once region was entered into the multiple regression model. Nonetheless, the deviations from that correlation are informative. The West region did not have a significantly elevated proportion of male births. Gujarati is a Group 1 language spoken predominantly in the West region, and Marathi and Konkani are Group 2 languages spoken mainly in the West region. The male birth proportion among native speakers of Group 1 or Group 2 languages in the West region was 0.518, compared to 0.491 among native speakers of other languages in the West ($p = 0.06$). Similarly, Bengali is a Group 1 language but falls into the East region. In West Bengal, the male birth proportion among Bengali native speakers is 0.509, compared to 0.528 among Hindi native speakers (also a Group 1 language) and 0.497 among native speakers of other languages ($p = 0.36$). Thus, culture may be the important construct rather than geographic location.

Women's labor force participation was hypothesized to be related to male birth proportion; nonetheless, it was not found to be associated with male birth in either the bivariate or multivariate analyses. Similarly, spatial exogamy, as measured by the timing of residence in current locality relative to timing of marriage, was not found to be associated with male birth.

The sex composition of surviving siblings was associated with male birth as hypothesized. Having no older brothers alive at approximately 20 weeks of gestation was associated with a higher proportion of male births from 1990 on, and having less than two older sisters was negatively correlated with male birth from the late 1980s onward. No significant interactions were found between number of surviving older brothers and birth order, between number of surviving older sisters and birth order, or between number of surviving older brothers and number of surviving older sisters. These findings indicate that parents who already had two or more daughters are more likely to have been using sex-selective abortion since the late 1980s to assure that the next child is a son. Similarly, parents with no sons are likely to have begun using this method to assure the birth of a son slightly later in the 1990s. This conclusion is consistent with other studies suggesting that, despite an overall preference for sons, parents in India desire a certain sex composition of offspring that includes one or two daughters (Das Gupta, 1987; Mishra et al., 2004; Pande, 2003).

The following capability factors were hypothesized to affect the ability to realize son preferences and to thus be associated with a higher proportion of male births: greater levels of education among both parents, greater wealth, and areas with greater access to medical technology. Although father's level of education was associated with male birth in the bivariate analysis, in the multivariate analysis, it was correlated with both mother's level of education and the asset index and thus did not retain statistical significance in the final model. Overall, mother's level of education at the middle school level had a greater magnitude and strength of association with male birth. However, when stratified by calendar year, women with a high school education showed a large rise in male birth proportion in the mid- to late-1990s. The most highly educated women appear to have just recently begun to utilize sex-selective abortion to control the sex composition of their family. It will be of interest to determine if data from the next round of the NFHS, due to be collected in 2005–2006, continues this trend. Physical proximity to towns was significantly associated with the proportion of male births, indicating that access is limited by distance from services.

During the interval from 1977–1999, no overall increase was observed over time in the proportion of births that were male. However, certain population subgroups did experience an increase. Families with no surviving sons showed an increase in the proportion of male births beginning in the 1990s, whereas families with two or more daughters showed an increase over time beginning slightly earlier—in the late 1980s. As noted above, mothers with a high school education showed a large increase in male births in the latter half of the 1990s, whereas mothers with a middle school level of education showed little change over time. These findings reflect a changing modality of control over family composition among those who have access to sex determination testing and abortion services and the resources to take advantage of them.

Chapter 6

The Effect of Prenatal Sex Selection on Gender Differentials in Mortality

The objective of this analysis is to investigate changes over time in gender differentials in infant and child mortality, and to determine if prenatal sex selection is having an effect on those differentials. As access to sex selection technology diffuses over time, if substitution is occurring, those with the highest propensity for sex selection should experience the lowest gender differentials. Girls born into families that practice prenatal selection are more likely to be wanted than girls born into families not practicing prenatal selection; thus, it is hypothesized that they will have lower levels of mortality, especially after the age of 1 year.

PROPENSITY SCORE

The logistic regression model of male birth proportion, developed in the previous chapter, was utilized to estimate a propensity score for each birth as the posterior predictive probability of male gender for an individual birth with a set of observed covariates. The propensity score represents how likely it is that a particular birth is a boy, given a set of background factors that may predispose toward prenatal selection. Adjustment for the propensity score not only provides an unbiased estimate of gender differentials in mortality in settings where prenatal sex selection is occurring, it also allows for comparison of gender differentials in mortality between children born to parents who are more and less likely to opt for sex selection and allows for comparisons over time, as prenatal sex selection has diffused.

The distribution of the propensity score for the 341,652 births is displayed in Figure 6.1. The mean propensity was 0.519 (range 0.473–0.577), and the median was 0.518 (IQR 0.511–0.525). In other words, the median predicted probability of a birth being male was 0.518, slightly higher than the naturally expected value of 0.513. The propensity score was categorized into five equal groups: the 1st quintile (Q1) ranged from 0.473–0.509, the 2nd (Q2) ranged from 0.509–0.516, the 3rd quintile (Q3) had values from 0.516–0.521, the 4rth (Q4) from 0.521–0.528, and the 5th quintile (Q5) ranged from 0.528–0.577. The ranges for the propensity quintiles may also be expressed as sex ratio at birth [$p / (1 - p)$]: Q1 corresponds to a low SRB of 0.90–1.04, Q2 to a natural SRB in the range 1.04–1.07, Q3 to a slightly elevated SRB of 1.07–1.09, Q4 to a moderately elevated SRB of 1.09–1.12, and Q5 to an extremely high SRB of 1.12–1.36.

Figure 6.1. Histogram of the propensity score for 341,652 births, India 1977–1999.

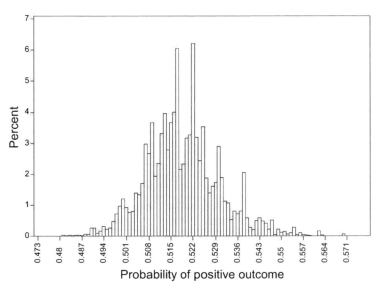

Table 6.1 displays the gender distribution of births within each propensity score quintile. The proportion of boys that fall into each quintile increases steadily from Q1 to Q5. The 1st quintile is composed of 50.5% boys and 49.5% girls, and the 5th quintile has 53.3% boys and 46.7% girls.

Figure 6.2 shows the distribution of propensity score quintiles over time. There is not much variation over time in the overall distribution, but when stratified by birth order and number and gender of surviving older siblings, as shown in Figure 6.3, patterns of sex selection emerge. Over time there is an increase in the proportion of births that fall into Q5, notably so among third

Table 6.1. Gender distribution within propensity score quintiles.

Propensity	Males		Females		Total
Quintile	Number	%	Number	%	Number
Q1	34,395	50.5%	33,756	49.5%	68,151
Q2	35,058	51.2%	33,359	48.8%	68,417
Q3	35,549	52.0%	32,783	48.0%	68,332
Q4	35,616	52.1%	32,782	47.9%	68,398
Q5	36,444	53.3%	31,910	46.7%	68,354
Total	177,062	51.8%	164,590	48.2%	341,652

Figure 6.2. Distribution of propensity score quintiles over time.

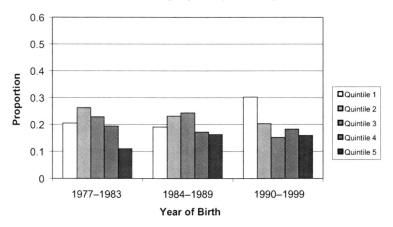

and fourth births with no surviving older brothers. Conversely, among second and higher order births with no surviving older sisters, there is an increase over time in the proportion of births falling into Q1, which indicates that in certain situations, girls are being selected as are boys.

Figure 6.3. Distribution of propensity score over time, by birth order and surviving older brothers.

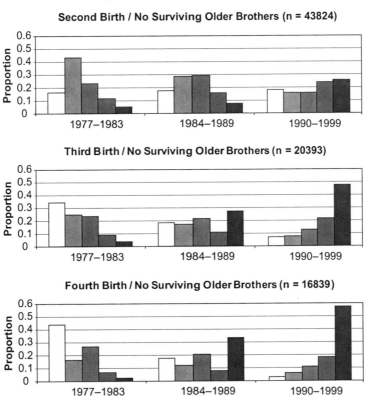

NEONATAL AND POSTNEONATAL MORTALITY

Infant mortality was segmented into deaths occurring in the neonatal period (up to 27 days after birth) and those occurring in the postneonatal period (28 days to 11 months after birth). In India, the predominant causes of neonatal mortality are low birth weight and infection, whereas the major causes of postneonatal mortality are diarrhea and acute respiratory infection.

The number of deaths by age at death, up to 60 months, show some heaping of age at death at 6, 12, 18, 24, 36, 48, and 60 months. Age at death was recorded in months up to age 36 months and in years after that. Due to this imprecise reporting of age at death, logistic regression analysis was used to analyze neonatal, postneonatal, and child mortality instead of a time to event analysis (survival analysis). Neonatal and postneonatal mortality rates are shown by child-level characteristics in Table 6.2, by family-level characteristics in Table 6.3, and by PSU-level characteristics in Table 6.4.

Child-Level Factors

As shown in Table 6.2, neonatal mortality (NNM) among births from 1977–1999 was 52.0 per 1,000 births and postneonatal mortality (PNM) was 30.6 per 1,000 births, which sum to an

Figure 6.4. Distribution of propensity score over time, by birth order and surviving older sisters.

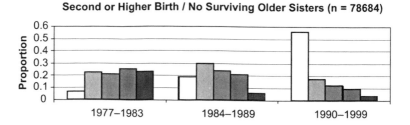

Table 6.2. Neonatal and postneonatal mortality by child-level characteristics.

Characteristic	Number of Births	Neonatal Mortality*	p-value	Postneonatal Mortality*	p-value
Overall	344,740	52.0	—	30.6	—
Gender:					
Male	178,684	55.7		28.7	
Female	166,056	48.1	<0.001	32.7	<0.001
Year of Birth (Quintiles):					
1977–1983	67,835	59.5		40.4	
1984–1986	69,484	55.0		34.1	
1987–1989	69,478	52.9		29.8	
1990–1992	68,758	48.8		25.7	
1993–1999	69,185	43.5	<0.001	22.8	<0.001
Multiple Births:					
No	339,886	48.4		29.8	
Yes	4,854	302.8	<0.001	85.7	<0.001
Preceding Birth Interval:					
N/A (First Birth)	89,969	60.4		27.2	
<24 Months	83,576	76.4		47.7	
24–35 Months	90,417	41.8		29.1	
36+ Months	80,775	27.8	<0.001	18.5	<0.001

(continued)

Table 6.2. Neonatal and postneonatal mortality by child-level characteristics. *(continued)*

Characteristic	Number of Births	Neonatal Mortality*	p-value	Postneonatal Mortality*	p-value
Mother's Age at Time of Birth:					
<20	82,125	68.9		34.2	
20–24	126,611	45.6		27.9	
25–29	82,424	42.9		28.3	
30–34	38,660	49.9		33.1	
35+	14,920	56.8	<0.001	37.8	<0.001
Birth Order:					
1	89,510	60.4		27.2	
2	81,657	46.8		27.3	
3	62,787	42.6		27.3	
4+	110,786	54.4	<0.001	37.5	<0.001
Number of Older Brothers Born:					
None	155,507	53.0		27.5	
One	103,050	46.2		28.0	
Two or More	86,183	57.0	<0.001	39.0	<0.001

Number of Older Sisters Born:					
None	155,503	55.4		28.1	
One	95,169	46.8		29.7	
Two or More	94,068	51.8	<0.001	35.7	<0.001
Surviving Older Brothers:					
None	171,229	58.4		29.6	
One	106,404	45.0		28.7	
Two or More	67,107	47.0	<0.001	36.1	<0.001
Surviving Older Sisters:					
None	168,917	59.4		30.3	
One	98,032	45.1		30.6	
Two or More	77,791	44.9	<0.001	31.3	0.55
Family Composition (Siblings):					
Birth Order 1:	97,512	60.4		27.2	
Birth Order 2:					
No Surviving Older Brothers	44,153	54.5		31.6	
One Surviving Older Brother	37,504	37.4		25.1	
Birth Order 3:					
No Surviving Older Brothers	20,553	52.6		31.4	
One Surviving Older Brother	30,287	40.7		27.6	
Two Surviving Older Brothers	11,947	29.5		26.0	

(continued)

Table 6.2. Neonatal and postneonatal mortality by child-level characteristics. *(continued)*

Characteristic	Number of Births	Neonatal Mortality*	p-value	Postneonatal Mortality*	p-value
Birth Order 4 or Higher					
No Surviving Older Brothers	17,013	64.7		44.0	
One Surviving Older Brothers	38,613	55.2		36.6	
Two or More Surviving Older Brothers	55,160	50.7	<0.001	40.4	<0.001
Propensity Score (Quintiles):					
Q1 = SRB 0.898–1.037	68,151	48.2		28.0	
Q2 = SRB 1.037–1.066	68,417	53.8		31.1	
Q3 = SRB 1.066–1.088	68,332	57.0		32.9	
Q4 = SRB 1.088–1.119	68,398	57.9		35.3	
Q5 = SRB 1.119–1.364	68,354	41.5	<0.001	24.9	<0.001

*per 1,000 live births.

Table 6.3. Neonatal and postneonatal mortality by family-level characteristics.

Characteristic	Number of Births	Neonatal Mortality*	p-value	Postneonatal Mortality*	p-value
Religion:					
Hindu	260,675	54.6		32.4	
Muslim	46,800	44.8		25.7	
Christian	21,280	29.8		17.3	
Other	15,819	36.8	<0.001	17.9	<0.001
Scheduled Caste/Tribe:					
Scheduled Caste	53,500	59.4		36.2	
Scheduled Tribe	47,836	52.9		34.1	
Neither	241,888	50.2	<0.001	28.9	<0.001
Household Standard of Living (Quintiles):					
Low	63,623	62.1		38.9	
Lower middle	70,674	57.1		37.0	
Middle	68,714	57.3		30.5	
Higher middle	71,384	46.4		27.1	
High	70,345	33.5	<0.001	16.4	<0.001

(continued)

Table 6.3. Neonatal and postneonatal mortality by family-level characteristics. *(continued)*

Characteristic	Number of Births	Neonatal Mortality*	p-value	Postneonatal Mortality*	p-value
Mother's Education:					
Illiterate	219,927	59.4		36.8	
< Middle School	63,865	41.0		21.7	
Middle School	24,613	37.4		15.1	
High School +	36,298	25.5	<0.001	10.2	<0.001
Father's Education:					
Illiterate	115,658	62.0		38.7	
< Middle School	94,250	52.6		31.2	
Middle School	45,225	46.5		28.4	
High School+	88,211	38.9	<0.001	18.8	<0.001
Mother's Labor Force Participation:					
None	215,633	50.2		28.8	
Noncash	50,486	57.4		34.3	
Cash	78,471	53.7	<0.001	33.2	<0.001

	N			
Mother's Residence Before Marriage:				
Lived here before marriage	130,379	49.5		28.5	
Moved here at marriage	117,356	52.6		30.6	
Moved here after marriage	97,005	54.6	0.001	33.5	<0.001
Mother Tongue:					
Group 1	204,533	55.8		33.1	
Group 2	18,190	40.1		18.8	
Group 4	46,410	44.6		22.9	
Other	75,558	50.1	<0.001	35.5	<0.001
Media Exposure:					
None	166,201	59.5		37.3	
One	93,571	48.8		26.9	
Two	70,082	39.1		19.6	
Three	14,886	34.6	<0.001	17.6	<0.001

*per 1,000 live births.

Table 6.4. Neonatal and postneonatal mortality by PSU-level characteristics.

Characteristic	Number of Births	Neonatal Mortality*	p-value	Postneonatal Mortality*	p-value
Urban/Rural Residence:					
Urban	93,995	36.9		20.8	
Rural	250,745	56.6	<0.001	33.6	<0.001
Region:					
Region 1: North	54,105	36.3		25.5	
Region 2: West	35,690	41.9		20.8	
Region 3: Central	129,773	60.9		37.8	
Region 4: East	31,430	53.6		30.9	
Region 5: Northeast	43,777	44.9		27.8	
Region 6: South	49,965	43.9	<0.001	22.5	<0.001
Predominant Mother Tongue:					
Group 1	204,299	55.9		33.4	
Group 2	18,575	39.3		18.6	
Group 4	47,410	44.5		22.8	
Other	74,456	50.5	<0.001	35.4	<0.001
Primary Health Center in Village:					
No	211,233	58.1		34.4	
Yes	32,289	46.0	<0.001	26.6	<0.001

	N	%	p-value	%	p-value
Nearest Hospital to Village (Quintiles):					
0–3 km	54,057	49.9		30.8	
4–7 km	49,257	59.0		33.8	
8–12 km	48,438	59.5		32.0	
13–21 km	42,941	58.3		34.7	
>22 km	49,606	56.7	<0.001	36.1	0.03
Mobile Health Unit in Village:					
No	203,814	55.7		32.5	
Yes	43,147	60.2	0.03	37.4	<0.001
Nearest Town to Village (Quintiles):					
0–5 km	53,121	53.4		31.2	
6–9 km	43,879	56.9		34.5	
10–14 km	46,393	56.6		31.4	
15–24 km	52,448	57.1		33.4	
>25 km	52,019	58.9	0.23	36.6	0.01
Electricity in Village:					
No	46,270	64.7		37.5	
Yes	200,881	54.4	<0.001	32.3	<0.001
Television in Village:					
No	36,177	61.8		37.4	
Yes	206,804	56.0	0.01	32.8	0.003

(continued)

Table 6.4. Neonatal and postneonatal mortality by PSU-level characteristics. *(continued)*

Characteristic	Number of Births	Neonatal Mortality*	p-value	Postneonatal Mortality*	p-value
Number of Households in Village (Quintiles):					
<125	47,070	59.8		37.7	
125–248	47,570	61.2		37.6	
249–400	49,144	55.3		32.6	
401–744	44,510	56.0		31.0	
745–8,930	47,874	50.0	<0.001	28.5	<0.001

Note. Nearly all of the rural PSUs were comprised of one village; however, 75 PSUs were comprised of two villages, and one PSU included three villages, hence the number of villages is slightly greater than the number of rural PSUs.

*per 1,000 live births.

infant mortality rate of 82.6 per 1,000. Neonatal mortality was lower among girls, as expected biologically, whereas postneonatal mortality was lower among boys. Girls had a neonatal mortality rate of 48.1 per 1,000 births, and boys had a rate 16% higher (55.7 per 1,000 births). On the other hand, postneonatal mortality was 14% higher among girls, 32.7 per 1,000, compared to 28.7 among boys. There was a significant and steady decline in both NNM and PNM over time from 1977 to 1999. Neonatal mortality declined 27% from 59.5 in 1977–1983 to 43.5 in 1993–1999. An even sharper decline of 44% was observed in postneonatal mortality, dropping from 40.4 in 1977–1983 to 22.8 in 1993–1999.

The highest mortality rates were observed among multiple births, with a NNM of 302.8 and PNM of 85.7 per 1,000. Shorter birth intervals were also associated with higher mortality. Children with birth intervals under 24 months had a NNM of 76.4 and a PNM of 47.7, followed by children with intervals from 24–36 months, with a NNM of 41.8 and a PNM of 29.1. A lower mortality was found among children with intervals of 36 months and greater, with a NNM of 27.8 and a PNM of 18.5. Neonatal mortality was higher among births to teenaged mothers (68.9), followed by children of mothers aged 35 and above (56.8), whereas postneonatal mortality was higher among births to older mothers aged 35 and above (37.8), followed by children of teenaged mothers (34.2).

By birth order, first births had the highest levels of NNM (60.4), reflecting biological causes, but those who survived the neonatal period had average levels of PNM (27.2), which were not notably higher than other birth orders. Fourth- and higher order births had elevated levels of both NNM (54.4) and

PNM (37.5), reflecting clustering of child deaths in families with replacement of prior deaths, a scarcity of resources in larger families, the higher risk characteristics of families with higher fertility, and the decline of fertility over time, along with mortality rates. When birth order was stratified by the number of surviving older brothers, the highest mortality rates were among high order births with no surviving older brothers. Indeed, within each birth order the highest mortality is among those with no surviving older brothers and declines steadily as the number of surviving older brothers increases, with the following exceptions: NNM was elevated (40.7) among third births with only one surviving older brother, and PNM was elevated (40.4) among fourth and higher births with two or more surviving older brothers.

When analyzed by propensity quintiles, both NNM and PNM rates were highest in the 4th quintile, corresponding to a moderately elevated sex ratio at birth of 1.09–1.12, followed by the 3rd quintile (SRB of 1.07–1.09), the 2nd quintile (a natural SRB of 1.04–1.07), and the 1st quintile (a low SRB of 0.90–1.04). Substantially lower mortality rates were observed in the 5th propensity score quintile (corresponding to a highly elevated SRB of 1.12–1.36), with a low NNM of 41.5, and a PNM of 24.9, likely reflecting the higher socioeconomic status of those who have the resources to practice sex-selective abortion.

Family-Level Factors

Hindu religion was associated with higher levels of both neonatal and postneonatal mortality, as was scheduled caste status, as shown in Table 6.3. Hindus had a NNM of 54.6, compared to 44.8 for Muslims, 29.8 for Christians, and 36.8 for other religions. The disparities by religion were not as great for PNM: 32.4 among births to Hindu families, 25.7 among Muslims, 17.3 among Christians, and 17.9 among families of other religions.

Mortality rates during the first year of life declined steadily as household standard of living increased, and as both mother's and father's level of education increased. NNM was 62.1 in the lowest standard of living quintile, nearly twice that in the highest standard of living quintile (33.5), whereas PNM in the lowest standard of living families (38.9) was more than twice the rate in the highest standard of living families (16.5). Similarly, for father's level of education, the NNM rates rose from 38.9 among children of high school graduates to 46.5 among infants of men who completed middle school to 62.0 among infants of illiterate men, and PNM rose from 18.8 among high school graduates to 38.7 among illiterates. The disparity in infant mortality rates was even greater by the mother's level of education. Births to illiterate mothers had a NNM of 59.4, compared to 41.0 for mothers with some education, 37.4 for mothers who completed middle school, and a low rate of 25.5 among births to high school graduates. An even wider gap was found for rates of PNM: 36.8 per 1,000 among births to illiterate mothers, compared to 10.2 among mothers who had a high school or greater education.

Infant mortality was higher among births to working mothers, especially those who did not receive cash in exchange for work, with a NNM of 57.4 and a PNM of 34.3. Rates were slightly lower among cash earners, with a NNM of 53.7 and a PNM of 33.2, and were even lower among women who did not work, with a NNM of 50.2 and a PNM of 28.8. Elevated rates were found among infants of women who practiced spatial exogamy, moving to their current place of residence at the time of marriage, with a NNM of 52.6 and a PNM of 30.6, compared to a NNM of 49.5 and a PNM of 28.5 among infants of women who lived in their current place of residence prior to their marriage. And even higher rates were observed among infants of women who moved to their current location at some point after marriage, with a NNM of 54.6 and a PNM of 33.5, perhaps reflecting risks of migration, including a lack of social capital or poorer socio-economic conditions among migrant populations.

Higher infant mortality was found in families with native languages falling into Group 1 (with a NNM of 55.8 and a PNM of 33.1) and "other" languages (with a NNM of 50.1 and a PNM of 35.5), whereas lower infant mortality rates were found among native speakers of Group 2 (with a NNM of 40.1 and a PNM of 18.8) and Group 4 (with a NNM of 44.6 and a PNM of 22.9) languages. Media exposure of mothers was measured by the number of the following media outlets that women were routinely exposed to: weekly television, weekly radio, and monthly visits to the cinema. Media exposure was related to both NNM and PNM, with rates declining as the number of media exposures increased. Infants of mothers who had no exposure to media had higher rates of NNM (59.5) and PNM (37.3), whereas those with one media outlet had a NNM of 48.8 and a PNM of 26.9, those with two media outlets had a NNM of 39.1 and a PNM of 19.6, and those with regular exposure to all three media types had a NNM of 34.6 and a PNM of 17.6.

PSU-Level Factors
Table 6.4 displays neonatal and postneonatal mortality by characteristics of the primary sampling unit, which in rural areas consisted of the village. Rural neonatal mortality rates were

50% higher than urban rates, 56.6 and 36.9, respectively, and rural postneonatal mortality (33.6) was 60% higher than that in urban areas (20.8). The Central and Eastern regions of the country had the highest infant mortality rates. Neonatal mortality reached 60.9 per 1,000 births, and postneonatal mortality reached 37.8 in the Central region of the country, composed of the least-developed states of India: Madhya Pradesh, Uttar Pradesh, Bihar, and Rajasthan. Elevated NNM (53.6) and PNM (30.9) also occurred in the Eastern region, which comprises the states of Orissa and West Bengal. The lowest NNM (36.3) was found in the more affluent Northern states of Haryana, New Delhi, Himachal Pradesh, Jammu, and Punjab, whereas the lowest PNM (22.5) occurred in the Southern states: Andhra Pradesh, Karnataka, Kerala, and Tamil Nadu. The mortality rates by the predominant mother tongue spoken in a PSU were similar to those for the family-level variable: lowest among Group 2 and Group 4 languages and higher among Group 1 and other languages. Villages without a primary health center (PHC) or nearby hospital had higher infant mortality. Neonatal mortality was 58.1 for births occurring in villages without a PHC and 46.0 in villages with a PHC, whereas PNM was 34.4 versus 26.6. Likewise, in villages without a hospital nearby, NNM ranged from 56.7 to 59.0, compared to 49.9 in villages with a hospital within 3 kilometers. PNM was not as strongly related to hospital proximity, ranging from 32.0 to 36.1 in villages more than 3 kilometers from a hospital versus 30.8 in villages closer to a hospital (p = 0.03). Villages with a mobile clinic had somewhat higher rates of mortality: neonatal mortality was 60.2 versus 55.7 in villages without a mobile clinic (p = 0.03), whereas PNM was 37.4 versus 32.5 in villages without a mobile clinic (p < 0.001). Distance to the nearest town was not related to NNM (p = 0.23), but it was related to PNM. Villages more than 25 kilometers from a town had higher postneonatal mortality (36.6) (p = 0.01). Villages with no electricity had higher mortality, with a PNM of 64.7 versus 54.4 and a NNM of 37.5 versus 32.3. Those villages without a single television had higher NNM (61.8) and PNM (37.4), and villages with fewer numbers of households had higher mortality. NNM was 59.8–61.2 in villages with fewer than 249 households, and PNM was 38 per 1,000 births.

Cʜɪʟᴅ Mᴏʀᴛᴀʟɪᴛʏ

Tables 6.5 through 6.7 display child mortality rates by individual, family, and PSU-level factors. The child mortality rate is defined as the number of deaths among children aged 12 months through 59 months divided by the number of children who survived to age 12 months. The overall child mortality in India among children born from 1977–1999 was 28.9 per 1,000 (note that those born 1994–1999 have censored data).

Child-Level Factors

The decline over time in child mortality was greater than that of infant mortality, as shown in Table 6.5, with a 58% drop from 41.0 per 1,000 in 1977–1983 to 17.1 per 1,000 in 1993–1999, reflecting improvements in immunization and health care, including oral rehydration therapy. Because lack of preventive and curative care is a major risk factor for child mortality, this is the stage when differential treatment of boys and girls is likely to have the greatest impact. Indeed, this is reflected in the gender-specific child

Table 6.5. Child mortality by child-level characteristics.

Characteristic	Number of 12-Month Olds	Child Mortality*	p-value
Overall	318,496	28.9	—
Gender:			
Male	164,762	23.6	
Female	153,734	34.5	<0.001
Year of Birth (Quintiles):			
1977–1983	61,706	41.0	
1984–1986	63,808	35.2	
1987–1989	64,173	30.6	
1990–1992	63,960	20.5	
1993–1999	64,849	17.1	<0.001
Multiple Births:			
No	315,407	28.7	
Yes	3,089	51.2	<0.001
Preceding Birth Interval:			
N/A (First Birth)	82,640	19.9	
<24 Months	74,051	47.7	
24–35 Months	84,542	32.0	
36+ Months	77,260	17.2	<0.001

(continued)

Table 6.5. Child mortality by child-level characteristics. *(continued)*

Characteristic	Number of 12-Month Olds	Child Mortality*	p-value
Subsequent Birth Interval:			
<24 Months	63,923	53.6	
24–35 Months	71,152	34.8	
36+ Months	57,164	29.8	
N/A (Last Birth)	126,255	12.6	<0.001
Mother's Age at Time of Birth:			
<20	73,936	30.5	
20–24	117,936	27.7	
25–29	77,171	27.8	
30–34	35,776	29.6	
35+	13,677	32.9	0.004
Birth Order:			
1	82,356	19.9	
2	76,130	25.2	
3	58,748	30.5	
4+	101,262	37.5	<0.001

Number of Older Brothers Born:			
None	144,028	22.6	
One	95,998	30.4	
Two or More	78,470	38.1	<0.001
Number of Older Sisters Born:			
None	143,647	23.5	
One	88,482	30.9	
Two or More	86,367	35.5	<0.001
Surviving Older Brothers:			
None	157,397	23.9	
One	99,164	31.2	
Two or More	61,935	37.5	<0.001
Surviving Older Sisters:			
None	155,046	24.8	
One	91,186	32.5	
Two or More	72,264	33.0	<0.001
Family Composition (Siblings):			
Birth Order 1	82,356	19.9	
Birth Order 2:			
No Surviving Older Brothers	40,749	24.8	
One Surviving Older Brother	35,381	25.6	

(continued)

Table 6.5. Child mortality by child-level characteristics. *(continued)*

Characteristic	Number of 12-Month Olds	Child Mortality*	p-value
Birth Order 3:			
No Surviving Older Brothers	18,947	29.3	
One Surviving Older Brother	28,434	32.1	
Two Surviving Older Brothers	11,367	28.8	
Birth Order 4 or Higher:			
No Surviving Older Brothers	15,345	35.6	
One Surviving Older Brothers	35,349	35.8	
Two or More Surviving Older Brothers	50,568	39.4	<0.001
Propensity Score (Quintiles):			
Q1 = SRB 0.898–1.037	63,096	24.4	
Q2 = SRB 1.037–1.066	62,901	27.4	
Q3 = SRB 1.066–1.088	62,639	35.1	
Q4 = SRB 1.088–1.119	62,816	33.5	
Q5 = SRB 1.119–1.364	64,228	24.3	<0.001

*per 1,000 children 12 months of age.

mortality rates, which are nearly 50% higher in girls than in boys: 34.5 versus 23.6 per 1,000, respectively, compared to 14% higher postneonatal mortality rates and 16% lower neonatal mortality rates in girls. Characteristics associated with child mortality are similar to those for neonatal and postneonatal mortality: multiple births, shorter birth intervals, mothers at either end of the reproductive age range at the time of birth, and fourth and higher birth order. The exceptions are those factors that lead to early mortality, such as low birth weight among first births, birth defects associated with late childbearing, and clustering of infant mortality within families, all of which are not risks for children who survive to the age of 12 months.

The relationship between child mortality and propensity score quintile was similar to that found for infant mortality: The lowest rates are observed at the extremes in the 1st and 5th quintiles, with rates of 24.4 and 24.3, respectively, followed by the 2nd quintile, at 27.4. The highest rates are found in the 3rd and 4th quintiles, 35.1 and 33.5, respectively. Infant mortality among births in the 5th quintile was much lower than any other quintile, but child mortality was also quite low in the 1st and 2nd quintiles as well as the 5th.

Family-Level Factors
Table 6.6 presents child mortality rates by family characteristics. Mortality was highest among Hindu families, at 30.3 per 1,000 children surviving to the age of 12 months, followed by Muslims (25.2), and was substantially lower among Christian families (15.8) and families of other religions (18.6). As was found for postneonatal mortality, scheduled castes and scheduled tribes had elevated mortality levels: 37.2 and 39.9, respectively.

Table 6.6. Child mortality by family-level characteristics.

Characteristic	Number of 12-Month Olds	Child Mortality*	p-value
Religion:			
Hindu	239,315	30.3	
Muslim	43,593	25.2	
Christian	20,443	15.8	
Other	14,994	18.6	<0.001
Scheduled Caste/Tribe:			
Scheduled Caste	48,699	37.2	
Scheduled Tribe	44,489	39.9	
Neither	223,932	25.4	<0.001
Household Standard of Living (Quintiles):			
Low	57,424	43.0	
Lower Middle	64,386	37.3	
Middle	63,126	31.0	
Higher Middle	66,515	19.1	
High	67,045	10.7	<0.001
Mother's Education:			
Illiterate	199,891	36.9	

			p-value
< Middle School	60,054	17.5	
Middle School	23,426	8.7	
High School+	35,090	4.5	<0.001
Father's Education:			
Illiterate	104,636	42.5	
< Middle School	86,773	28.4	
Middle School	42,170	22.0	
High School+	83,638	13.0	<0.001
Mother's Labor Force Participation:			
None	199,918	24.8	
Noncash	46,256	35.7	
Cash	72,194	35.8	<0.001
Mother's Residence Here Before Marriage:			
Lived Here Before Marriage	121,014	28.0	
Moved Here at Marriage	108,377	28.4	
Moved Here After Marriage	89,105	30.8	0.014

(continued)

Table 6.6. Child mortality by family-level characteristics. *(continued)*

Number of Characteristic	Child 12-Month Olds	Mortality*	p-value
Mother Tongue:			
Group 1	187,447	33.1	
Group 2	17,266	17.7	
Group 4	43,461	19.6	
Other	70,280	27.2	<0.001
Media Exposure:			
None	150,885	38.7	
One	87,116	22.4	
Two	66,350	14.6	
Three	14,145	11.2	<0.001

*per 1,000 children 12 months of age.

Table 6.7. Child mortality by PSU-level characteristics.

Characteristic	Number of 12-Month Olds	Child Mortality*	p-value
Urban/Rural Residence:			
Urban	88,769	16.9	<0.001
Rural	229,727	32.6	
Region:			
Region 1: North	50,868	17.0	
Region 2: West	33,607	20.2	
Region 3: Central	117,329	39.0	
Region 4: East	28,604	22.0	
Region 5: Northeast	41,265	29.6	
Region 6: South	46,823	19.5	<0.001
Predominant Mother Tongue:			
Group 1	187,110	33.4	
Group 2	17,634	17.4	
Group 4	44,399	19.9	
Other	69,353	25.7	<0.001
Primary Health Center in Village:			
No	192,983	33.3	
Yes	30,126	26.2	<0.001

(continued)

Table 6.7. Child mortality by PSU-level characteristics. *(continued)*

Characteristic	Number of 12-Month Olds	Child Mortality*	p-value
Mobile Health Unit in Village:			
No	187,048	32.3	0.47
Yes	39,235	33.6	
Nearest Hospital to Village (Quintiles):			
0–3 km	50,065	29.0	
4–7 km	45,024	33.1	
8–12 km	44,266	32.7	
13–21 km	39,156	34.4	
>22 km	45,304	33.7	0.06
Nearest Town to Village (Quintiles):			
0–5 km	49,078	29.9	
6–9 km	40,190	32.7	
10–14 km	42,519	31.7	
15–24 km	47,902	33.1	
>25 km	47,408	35.3	0.07
Electricity in Village:			
No	41,794	41.9	
Yes	184,654	30.0	<0.001

Television in Village:			
No	32,826	43.6	
Yes	189,768	30.9	<0.001
Number of Households in Village (Quintiles):			
<125	43,034	37.2	
125–248	43,306	35.2	
249–400	45,019	33.0	
401–744	40,849	30.6	
745–8,930	44,331	26.8	<0.001

*per 1,000 children 12 months of age.

Greater disparities by standard of living status were found for child mortality than for either NNM or PNM. In the lowest standard of living quintile compared to the highest standard of living quintile, neonatal mortality was 85% higher, postneonatal mortality was more than twice as high, and child mortality was four times higher: 43.0 versus 10.7. Similar disparities were found by father's level of education. Child mortality was 13.0 among children of high school educated fathers, 22.0 among middle school educated fathers, 28.4 among fathers with some education, and 42.5 among children of illiterate fathers. Even greater disparities were found by mother's level of education: 4.5 among children of mothers with a high school education, 8.7 among middle school educated mothers, 17.5 for mothers with some education, and more than double that among the majority of mothers with no education (36.9). The result is an 8-fold gap in child mortality rates between mothers with high school education and illiterate mothers.

Children of working mothers had higher mortality levels (35.7–35.8) compared to nonworking mothers (24.8), regardless of cash-earning status. Rates did not vary much by whether the mother lived in the current place of residence before marriage (28.0), moved there at the time of marriage (28.4), or moved there at some point after marriage (30.8). By native tongue, Group 2 and Group 4 languages were associated with lower rates (17.7 and 19.6, respectively), and Group 1 (33.1) and other languages (27.2) were associated with higher child mortality rates, as was found for infant mortality. Greater levels of media exposure were associated with lower levels of child mortality. Children of women with no regular exposure to radio, television, or cinema had a mortality of 38.7, whereas those with one source of media had a rate of 22.4, with two media sources the rate was 14.6, and with exposure to all three sources of media, a low rate of 11.2.

PSU-Level Factors

Table 6.7 examines child mortality rates by characteristics of the primary sampling unit, that is, the village or census block. Child mortality in rural areas was 32.6 per 1,000 children who survived to the age of 12 months, nearly double the rate found for rural areas, 16.9. This rural/urban gap was wider than that found for neonatal or postneonatal mortality, with rural neonatal mortality 54% higher than urban and with rural postneonatal mortality 61% higher than urban.

As in the case of infant mortality, the central region of the country had the worst child mortality rate: 39.0. However, the Eastern region, which had the second highest infant mortality, faired relatively better in child mortality, with a rate of 22.0. The Northeastern states had the second highest child mortality rate of 29.6. The remaining regions had lower rates of 20.2 and 19.5 in the West and South, and as with infant mortality, the more prosperous states in the North had the lowest rate of 17.0. Reflecting these regional differences, rates were lowest in clusters where the Group 2 (17.4) and Group 4 (19.9) native languages predominated, higher where the "other" languages predominated, at 25.7, and highest in the areas where the Group 1 native tongues were dominant (33.4).

Mortality was elevated in villages lacking a primary health center (33.3) but did not vary greatly by proximity to a hospital, ranging from 29.9 to 34.4 (p = 0.06), or by the presence of a mobile health unit (p = 0.47). Child mortality was elevated in villages with no electricity (41.9), no television (43.6), and with fewer households (35.2–37.2).

CHANGES OVER TIME IN GENDER DIFFERENTIALS BY PROPENSITY SCORE

The hypothesis of interest is whether sex-selective abortion is substituting for neonatal, postneonatal, or child mortality. The hypothesis was tested using the propensity for sex selection as a proxy measure of sex-selective abortion. If excess female mortality declined disproportionately in the high propensity quintiles over time, then that would provide evidence that sex selection is substituting for infant and child mortality.

First, the data were examined in a contingency table analysis of gender differentials in mortality by propensity score, and gender differentials by year of birth and propensity score. Odds ratios for female versus male mortality were calculated as a *relative* measure of the gender differential. Next, the rates were graphed by gender, year of birth, and propensity score to examine the change in gender-specific mortality patterns. Area under the curve (AUC) was calculated using the linear trapezoidal method and the difference in AUC between boys and girls was computed for each propensity score quintile over time to examine the change in the *absolute* gender differential in mortality over time. Finally, a multivariate regression model for each of the three stages of mortality (neonatal, postneonatal, and child) was developed to determine if there were an independent, statistically significant interaction between gender, year of birth, and propensity score.

Table 6.8 displays odds ratios (OR) and 95% confidence intervals (CI) for female versus male mortality for births in the interval from 1977–1999, overall and by propensity score quintile. Overall, the odds of neonatal mortality among girls were 86% of that among boys (OR 0.86, 95% CI 0.82–0.89). The odds ratio increased as the propensity increased, from 0.79 in Q1 to 0.99 in Q5. Among births in the highest propensity quintile there was no difference in neonatal mortality between girls and boys (OR 0.99, 95% CI 0.89–1.10, p = 0.85).

In the postneonatal period, overall, girls were 15% more likely to die than boys (OR 1.15, 95% CI 1.09–1.21). However, in the lower propensity quintiles, there was no significant difference between female and male mortality. The odds ratio increased as propensity increased: the OR was not significantly different than unity in the 1st propensity quintile (OR 0.98, 95% CI 0.89–1.09, p = 0.76) or in the 2nd quintile (OR 1.07, 95% CI 0.97–1.19, p = 0.18), but the OR was significantly elevated in the 3rd through 5th quintiles, with values of 1.24 in the 3rd, 1.18 in the 4th, and 1.40 (95% CI 1.24–1.59) in the 5th propensity quintile.

For child mortality, female mortality was significantly higher than male mortality in each of the propensity quintiles, but the magnitude of the female excess increased as the propensity increased from 20% in the lowest propensity quintile to 72% in the highest propensity quintile.

Tables 6.9 to 6.11 present the same analysis but for different time periods. Table 6.9 covers the period before sex-selective abortion was available (1977–1983), Table 6.10 includes births from the mid- to late-1980s, when the use of sex-selective abortion was just beginning to diffuse, and Table 6.11 presents

Table 6.8. Neonatal, postneonatal, and child mortality by gender and propensity score quintile, India, 1977–1999.

Propensity Quintile/Gender	Number of Births	Neonatal Mortality[1]	OR[2] (95% CI[3])	p-value	Postneonatal Mortality[1]	OR[2] (95% CI[3])	p-value	Number of 12-Month-Olds	Child Mortality	OR[2] (95% CI[3])	p-value
Overall:											
Male	178,684	55.7	0.86 (0.82–0.89)	<0.001	28.7	1.15 (1.09–1.21)	<0.001	164,762	23.6	1.48 (1.40–1.56)	<0.001
Female	166,056	48.1			32.7			153,734	34.5		
Q1:											
Male	34,395	53.5	0.79 (0.73–0.86)	<0.001	28.2	0.98 (0.89–1.09)	0.76	31,644	22.3	1.20 (1.07–1.35)	0.002
Female	33,756	42.8			27.8			31,452	26.6		
Q2:											
Male	35,058	58.9	0.81 (0.75–0.88)	<0.001	30.1	1.07 (0.97–1.19)	0.18	32,106	23.5	1.35 (1.21–1.50)	<0.001
Female	33,359	48.4			32.2			30,795	31.4		
Q3:											
Male	35,549	60.3	0.88 (0.81–0.95)	0.002	29.6	1.24 (1.11–1.38)	<0.001	32,568	26.9	1.66 (1.50–1.83)	<0.001
Female	32,783	53.4			36.4			30,071	43.9		
Q4:											
Male	35,616	61.4	0.87 (0.81–0.95)	0.001	32.5	1.18 (1.06–1.32)	0.002	32,640	26.1	1.62 (1.45–1.82)	<0.001
Female	32,782	54.1			38.3			30,176	41.6		
Q5:											
Male	36,444	41.7	0.99 (0.89–1.10)	0.85	21.0	1.40 (1.24–1.59)	<0.001	34,323	18.3	1.72 (1.50–1.97)	<0.001
Female	31,910	41.3			29.3			29,905	31.1		

[1]per 1,000 live births. [2]OR = odds ratio. [3]CI = confidence interval.

Table 6.9. Neonatal mortality by year of birth, propensity score quintile, and gender, India, 1977–1999.

Propensity Quintile/ Gender	1977–1983			1984–1989			1990–1999		
	Number of Births	Neonatal Mortality[1]	OR[2] (95% CI[3])	Number of Births	Neonatal Mortality[1]	OR[2] (95% CI[3])	Number of Births	Neonatal Mortality[1]	OR[2] (95% CI[3])
Overall:									
Male	35,156	65.7	0.79 (0.73–0.86)	72,039	57.4	0.87 (0.82–0.92)	71,489	48.9	0.88 (0.83–0.94)
Female	32,679	52.8***		66,923	50.3***		66,454	43.4***	
Q1:									
Male	5,686	50.1	0.74 (0.61–0.89)	10,526	66.0	0.78 (0.69–0.89)	18,183	46.5	0.82 (0.72–0.94)
Female	5,740	37.3**		10,200	52.3***		17,816	38.6**	
Q2:									
Male	7,961	69.6	0.78 (0.68–0.91)	14,106	56.1	0.80 (0.70–0.91)	12,991	55.2	0.86 (0.75–0.99)
Female	7,454	55.2**		13,426	45.2***		12,479	47.9*	
Q3:									
Male	7,771	67.9	0.85 (0.72–0.99)	17,138	63.5	0.92 (0.82–1.03)	10,640	49.4	0.82 (0.70–0.97)
Female	7,131	58.1*		15,983	58.8		9,669	41.0*	
Q4:									
Male	7,347	76.9	0.81 (0.68–0.96)	14,505	55.1	0.87 (0.75–1.01)	13,764	59.0	0.93 (0.81–1.06)
Female	6,696	62.9*		13,221	48.4		12,865	55.0	
Q5:									
Male	5,868	61.1	0.82 (0.66–1.03)	15,121	43.4	1.02 (0.87–1.19)	15,455	33.2	1.06 (0.91–1.24)
Female	5,251	50.9		13,490	44.1		13,169	35.0	

[1]per 1,000 live births. [2]OR = odds ratio. [3]CI = confidence interval.
*p < 0.05. **p < 0.01. ***p < 0.001.

Table 6.10. Postneonatal mortality by year of birth, propensity score quintile, and gender, India, 1977–1999.

Propensity Quintile/ Gender	1977–1983			1984–1989			1990–1999		
	Number of Births	Post-neonatal Mortality[1]	OR[2] (95% CI[3])	Number of Births	Post-neonatal Mortality[1]	OR[2] (95% CI[3])	Number of Births	Post-neonatal Mortality[1]	OR[2] (95% CI[3])
Overall:									
Male	35,156	39.3	1.20 (1.09–1.32)	72,039	31.5	1.16 (1.08–1.25)	71,489	24.7	1.06 (0.98–1.16)
Female	32,679	46.8***		66,923	36.3***		66,454	26.2	
Q1:									
Male	5,686	33.4	1.08 (0.87–1.34)	10,526	31.2	0.97 (0.81–1.15)	18,183	27.6	0.93 (0.80–1.08)
Female	5,740	36.0		10,200	30.2		17,816	25.8	
Q2:									
Male	7,961	42.3	1.10 (0.91–1.33)	14,106	30.7	1.10 (0.93–1.30)	12,991	26.7	0.98 (0.81–1.18)
Female	7,454	46.4		13,426	33.6		12,479	26.1	
Q3:									
Male	7,771	35.9	1.34 (1.09–1.66)	17,138	35.0	1.13 (0.97–1.30)	10,640	22.7	1.34 (1.08–1.66)
Female	7,131	47.8**		15,983	39.2		9,669	30.2**	
Q4:									
Male	7,347	47.8	1.29 (1.04–1.60)	14,505	34.0	1.26 (1.08–1.48)	13,764	28.2	0.99 (0.82–1.18)
Female	6,696	60.9*		13,221	42.5**		12,865	27.9	
Q5:									
Male	5,868	34.3	1.25 (0.96–1.63)	15,121	24.7	1.45 (1.21–1.75)	15,455	14.9	1.42 (1.13–1.77)
Female	5,251	42.6		13,490	35.6**		13,169	21.0**	

[1]per 1,000 live births. [2]OR = odds ratio. [3]CI = confidence interval.
*p < 0.05 **p < 0.01 ***p < 0.001

Table 6.11. Child mortality by year of birth, propensity score quintile, and gender, India, 1977–1999.

Propensity Quintile/ Gender	Year of Birth								
	1977–1983			1984–1989			1990–1999		
	Number of 1-Year Olds	Child Mortality[1]	OR[2] (95% CI[3])	Number of 1-Year Olds	Child Mortality[1]	OR[2] (95% CI[3])	Number of 1-Year Olds	Child Mortality[1]	OR[2] (95% CI[3])
Overall:									
Male	31,888	32.6	1.56 (1.41–1.72)	66,257	27.9	1.39 (1.29–1.50)	66,617	14.8	1.57 (1.42–1.73)
Female	29,818	49.9***		61,724	38.3***		62,192	23.0***	
Q1:									
Male	5,231	32.1	1.16 (0.92–1.47)	9,528	24.8	1.16 (0.95–1.41)	16,885	17.3	1.26 (1.05–1.50)
Female	5,333	37.2		9,390	28.6		16,729	21.7**	
Q2:									
Male	7,159	33.0	1.32 (1.08–1.61)	12,972	23.6	1.37 (1.16–1.62)	11,975	17.2	1.35 (1.09–1.68)
Female	6,755	43.1**		12,445	32.1***		11,595	23.2**	
Q3:									
Male	7,036	30.1	2.03 (1.65–2.50)	15,607	32.4	1.37 (1.18–1.58)	9,925	15.9	2.08 (1.67–2.59)
Female	6,479	59.3***		14,557	43.8		9,035	32.6***	
Q4:									
Male	6,602	38.4	1.78 (1.43–2.21)	13,363	32.8	1.47 (1.25–1.73)	12,675	12.9	1.84 (1.45–2.35)
Female	6,032	66.4***		12,201	47.5***		11,943	23.6***	
Q5:									
Male	5,383	26.2	1.79 (1.32–2.42)	14,198	25.2	1.65 (1.38–1.98)	14,742	8.7	1.86 (1.40–2.46)
Female	4,840	45.9***		12,590	40.9***		12,475	16.0***	

[1]per 1,000 children surviving to age 12 months. [2]OR = odds ratio. [3]CI = confidence interval.
*p < 0.05. **p < 0.01. ***p < 0.001.

the mortality experience of births in the 1990s, when use of sex-selective abortion was more widespread.

The gender gap (male excess) in neonatal mortality narrowed over time from a relative odds of female mortality of 0.79 in 1977–1983 to 0.87 in 1984–1989 to 0.88 in 1990–1999. In the early time period before sex selection was available, even in the high propensity quintile (Q5), girls had lower neonatal mortality than boys (OR 0.82, 95% CI 0.66–1.03), as shown in Table 6.9; however, over time it increased to 1.02 (95% CI 0.87–1.19) in the late 1980s and then to 1.06 (95% CI 0.91–1.24) in 1990s, as shown in Tables 6.10 and 6.11, respectively. The odds ratio increased to a lesser extent over time within most of the other propensity quintiles. In the 4th quintile (Q4) the OR increased from 0.81 in the late 1970s/early 1980s to 0.87 in the late 1980s and to 0.93 in the 1990s, and in the 2nd quintile (Q2), the OR increased from 0.78 to 0.80 in the late 1980s to 0.86 in 1990s. Similarly, in the lowest propensity quintile (Q1) the OR increased from 0.74 in 1977–1983 to 0.78 in 1984–1989 and to 0.82 in 1990–1999. In the 3rd propensity quintile, the change in the gender differential showed a different pattern over time, with an initial decline in the gap, followed by an increase; the OR increased from 0.85 in 1977–1984 to 0.92 in the late 1980s, then back down to 0.82 in the 1990s.

The excess in female postneonatal mortality declined over time from 20% (p < 0.001) in the late 1970s/early 1980s to 16% (p < 0.001) in the late 1980s, to a nonsignificant level of 6% in the 1990s (p = 0.17). Among infants in the two lower propensity quintiles, the gender differential in postneonatal mortality was not significantly elevated in any of the time periods. Within Q1 the OR in 1977–1983 was 1.08 (p = 0.49), in 1984–1989 it was

0.97 (p = 0.70), and in 1990–1999 it was 0.93 (p = 0.37). In Q2 the OR was 1.10 (p = 0.31) in 1977–1983 and remained at 1.10 (p = 0.27) in 1984–1989, and it declined to 0.98 (p = 0.82) in 1990–1999. The 3rd propensity quintile (Q3) again showed an initial decline in the OR from 1.34 (p = 0.01) in the early years to 1.13 (p = 0.11) in the late 1980s and climbed again to 1.34 (p = 0.01) in the 1990s. The 4th quintile showed no change in the gender differential from 1977–1983 to 1984–1989, with ORs of 1.29 (p = 0.02) and 1.26 (p = 0.004) and then showed a sharp decline to 0.99 (p = 0.90) in 1990–1999. The highest propensity quintile (Q5) was the only one where female postneonatal mortality remained consistently elevated above that of males and increased over time. Girls had 25% higher postneonatal mortality in 1977–1983 (OR 1.25, p = 0.10), increasing to 45% in 1984–1989 (OR 1.45, p < 0.001) and remaining at that level in 1990–1999 (OR 1.42, p = 0.002).

The excess of female child mortality initially declined from 56% in the early period (1977–1983) to 39% in the mid- to late 1980s but jumped back up again in the 1990s to 57%. The ORs in the two lowest propensity quintiles changed little over time. In the 1st quintile the OR for female versus male child mortality was initially 1.16 (p = 0.21), remained at 1.16 (p = 0.14) in 1984–1989, and increased slightly to 1.26 (p = 0.01) in 1990–1999. The odds ratios in the 2nd propensity quintile remained significantly elevated at a constant level of 1.32 to 1.37 over the three time periods. The 3rd propensity quintile showed a sharp decline in the gender differential in child mortality from the late 1970s/early 1980s (OR 2.03, 95% CI 1.65–2.50) to the mid- to late-1980s (OR 1.37, 95% CI 1.18–1.58), but the relative difference increased again in the 1990s to the previous level (OR 2.08,

95% CI 1.67–2.59). A similar pattern was observed in the two highest propensity quintiles, although the initial decline was not as striking as that in Q3. The initial odds ratios, 1.78 ($p < 0.001$) and 1.79 ($p < 0.001$) in Q4 and Q5, respectively, declined to 1.47 ($p < 0.001$) and 1.65 ($p < 0.001$) in the mid- to late-1980s and then rose again in the 1990s to 1.84 ($p < 0.001$) and 1.86 ($p < 0.001$).

To summarize, it appears from this preliminary analysis, which is not adjusted for changes in other risk factors over time, that sex-selective abortion is not substituting for neonatal mortality. In fact, the opposite is occurring: the relative survival of female neonates is worsening among those most likely to utilize sex-selective abortion. The situation is slightly different for postneonatal mortality. Among those with an extreme propensity for sex selection of males, the relative survival of females has worsened over time, but among those with a moderate propensity, female survival has improved. The time trend in female excess child mortality is not continuous. There was an initial decline in the mid- to late 1980s among those with a propensity for sex selection, indicating that substitution was occurring, but in the 1990s that trend was reversed, with an upturn in excess female mortality among those with a greater propensity for sex selection of males.

Absolute Gender Difference

The odds ratio analysis provides information on the *relative* gap between female and male mortality levels. The area under the mortality curves was analyzed in order to examine changes over time in the *absolute* gender differences. Figure 6.5 displays the male and female neonatal mortality curves by propensity quintile over time, and Table 6.12 shows the AUC and the

Figure 6.5. Neonatal mortality by year of birth, propensity score quintile, and gender.

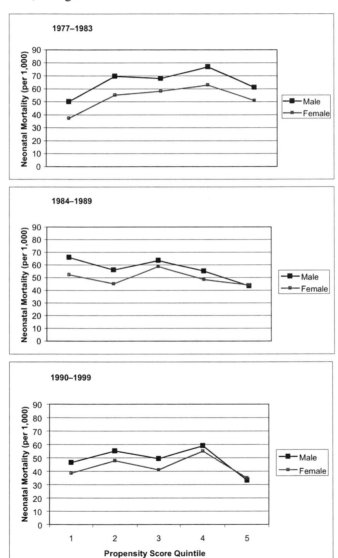

Table 6.12. Area under the neonatal mortality curve by year of birth and propensity score.

Year of Birth	Propensity	AUC Male	AUC Female	Difference Female-Male	% of Total
1977–1983					
	Q1–Q2	59.9	46.3	–13.6	27.4%
	Q2–Q3	68.8	56.7	–12.1	24.3%
	Q3–Q4	72.4	60.5	–11.9	23.9%
	Q4–Q5	69.0	56.9	–12.1	24.3%
	Total			–49.7	
1984–1989					
	Q1–Q2	61.1	48.8	–12.3	42.7%
	Q2–Q3	59.8	52.0	–7.8	27.1%
	Q3–Q4	59.3	53.6	–5.7	19.8%
	Q4–Q5	49.3	46.3	–3.0	10.4%
	Total			–28.8	
1990–1999					
	Q1–Q2	50.9	43.3	–7.6	33.4%
	Q2–Q3	52.3	44.5	–7.8	34.5%
	Q3–Q4	54.2	48.0	–6.2	27.3%
	Q4–Q5	46.1	45.0	–1.1	4.8%
	Total			–22.8	

difference in AUC (female-male), which corresponds to the area lying between the two curves. The AUC difference or absolute gender gap declined over time from –49.7 in 1977–1983 to –28.8 in 1984–1989 to –22.8 in 1990–1999. The negative sign indicates that male mortality was higher than female mortality; thus, the decline signifies a worsening of female neonatal mortality vis-à-vis male mortality. In the earliest time period, prior to the use of sex selection, the gap was evenly distributed between the propensity quintiles: 27% of the area fell between propensity quintiles Q1 and Q2, 24% fell between Q2 and Q3, 24% fell between Q3 and Q4, and 24% fell between Q4 and Q5. Over time, the negative gap shifted to the lower propensity quintiles: in 1984–1989, 43% fell between Q1 and Q2, 27% fell between Q2 and Q3, 20% fell between Q3 and Q4, and 10% fell between Q4 and Q5. And the gap shifted even further in the 1990s, with 33% between Q1 and Q2, 35% between Q2 and Q3, 27% between Q3 and Q4, and only 5% between Q4 and Q5. These data suggest that sex-selective abortion is not substituting for neonatal mortality; indeed, they appear to be complementing each other.

Figure 6.6 and Table 6.13 display the gender-specific post-neonatal mortality curves and AUC difference. The absolute gender gap in postneonatal mortality declined over time from 34.6 in the late 1970s/early 1980s to 20.6 in the mid- to late-1980s and down to 8.8 in the 1990s. The distribution by propensity quintile did not change much over time. In the early period, before sex-selective abortion was available, those with the highest propensity for sex selection had the greatest gender gap in postneonatal mortality: a total of 67% in the two highest quintiles. Over time, as sex selection began to be used in the mid- to late-1980s, the proportion of the gender gap in the two highest quintiles increased slightly to 78%, whereas the proportion in the two lowest quintiles dropped from 33% to 22%. In the 1990s, as sex selection diffused more widely, the distribution did not change greatly: In the lowest quintiles the proportion remained at 26% (with a male excess at the very lowest quintile), and the proportion remained at 74% in the two highest

Figure 6.6. Postneonatal mortality by year of birth, propensity score quintile, and gender.

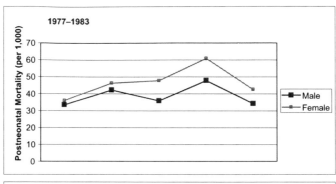

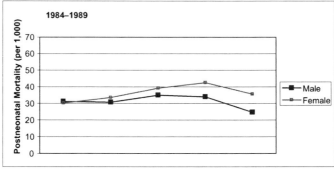

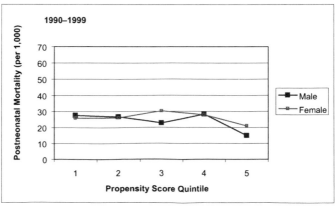

Table 6.13. Area under the postneonatal mortality curve by year of birth and propensity score.

Year of Birth	Propensity	AUC Male	AUC Female	Difference Female-Male	% of Total
1977–1983					
	Q1–Q2	37.9	41.2	3.4	9.7%
	Q2–Q3	39.1	47.1	8.0	23.2%
	Q3–Q4	41.9	54.4	12.5	36.2%
	Q4–Q5	41.1	51.8	10.7	31.0%
	Total			34.6	
1984–1989					
	Q1–Q2	31.0	31.9	0.9	4.6%
	Q2–Q3	32.9	36.4	3.6	17.3%
	Q3–Q4	34.5	40.9	6.4	30.9%
	Q4–Q5	29.4	39.1	9.7	47.2%
	Total			20.6	
1990–1999					
	Q1–Q2	27.2	26.0	–1.2	–13.7%
	Q2–Q3	24.7	28.2	3.5	39.4%
	Q3–Q4	25.5	29.1	3.6	41.1%
	Q4–Q5	21.6	24.5	2.9	33.1%
	Total			8.8	

quintiles. These data indicate that sex-selective abortion has not been substituting for postneonatal mortality, but there also does not appear to be as much of an additive effect as there was with neonatal mortality.

Child mortality curves are shown in Figure 6.7, and AUC differences are shown in Table 6.14. The absolute gender difference in child mortality dropped by 50% over time, declining from 79.7 in 1977–1983, to 44.4 in 1984–1989, to 39.3 in

Figure 6.7. Child mortality by year of birth, propensity score quintile, and gender.

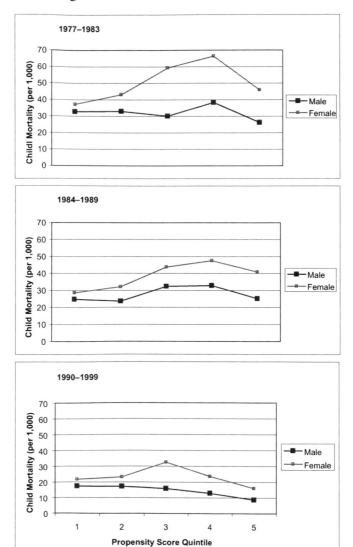

Table 6.14. Area under the child mortality curve by year of birth and propensity score.

Year of Birth	Propensity	AUC Male	AUC Female	Difference Female-Male	% of Total
1977–1983					
	Q1–Q2	32.6	40.2	7.6	9.5%
	Q2–Q3	31.6	51.2	19.7	24.7%
	Q3–Q4	34.3	62.9	28.6	35.9%
	Q4–Q5	32.3	56.2	23.9	29.9%
	Total			79.7	
1984–1989					
	Q1–Q2	24.2	30.4	6.2	13.9%
	Q2–Q3	28.0	38.0	10.0	22.4%
	Q3–Q4	32.6	45.7	13.1	29.4%
	Q4–Q5	29.0	44.2	15.2	34.3%
	Total			44.4	
1990–1999					
	Q1–Q2	17.3	22.5	5.2	13.2%
	Q2–Q3	16.6	27.9	11.4	28.9%
	Q3–Q4	14.4	28.1	13.7	34.9%
	Q4–Q5	10.8	19.8	9.0	22.9%
	Total			39.3	

1990–1999. The proportion of the gender gap that fell in the lower propensity quintiles increased somewhat over time from 34% to 36% to 42%, with a corresponding decline in the upper propensity quintiles from 66% to 64% to 58%. The bulk of the decline occurred in the highest propensity quintile: from 30% in 1977–1983 down to 23% in the 1990s. These data indicate that some substitution of sex-selective abortion for child mortality may have been occurring.

Mᴜʟᴛɪᴠᴀʀɪᴀᴛᴇ Aɴᴀʟʏsᴇs

The substitution hypothesis was tested in the multivariate models by a three-way interaction term between year of birth, gender, and propensity score. Formally stated, the hypothesis to be tested in the multivariate analyses is as follows:

> H_A: In the later calendar years (1984–1989 and 1990–1999), girls in the upper propensity score quintiles (Q4 and Q5) will have progressively lower mortality relative to boys than they did in the earliest time period (1977–1983), and the decline will be greater than that among girls in the lower propensity score quintiles.

If the interaction term between the dummy variables for year of birth 1990–1999, gender, and Q5 is statistically significant and negatively signed, that will provide evidence that prenatal selection is substituting for child mortality. Further, if the interaction term between the dummy variables for year of birth 1984–1989, gender, and Q5 is also negatively signed but of a lesser magnitude than the prior interaction term, that will provide evidence that there has been a progressive decline over time in girls' relative mortality in the high propensity quintile. Similar interactions will be assessed for year of birth, gender, and Q4, the 4th propensity quintile.

Neonatal Mortality

Multilevel logistic regression analysis was performed on the neonatal mortality data. Individual child-level factors (Level 1), family-level factors (Level 2), and PSU-level (Level 3) factors were included in the regression model. The intraclass correlation

(ICC or ρ) is the proportion of total residual variance attributable to a particular level. For the random intercept (variance components) model with no covariates, it is estimated as $(\tau_{00} + \tau_{11})/(\tau_{00} + \tau_{11} + \sigma_e^2)$, where s_e^2 (the variance of the individual-level error) may be estimated for binary data as $\pi^2/3 = 3.29$ (Snijders & Bosker, 1999). At the family level, $\rho_f = (1.637 + 0.237)/(1.637 + 0.237 + 3.29) = 0.363$. This indicates that 36% of the residual variance in neonatal mortality is attributable to family. The residual variance attributable to Level 3 (PSU) is: $\rho_p = 0.237/(1.637 + 0.237 + 3.29) = 0.046$. These results are consistent with prior studies finding clustering of adverse reproductive outcomes within families (Arulampalam & Bhalotra, 2006; Louis et al., 2005). The probability of neonatal mortality in the unadjusted model is $\exp(-3.069)/[1 + \exp(-3.069)] = 0.044$. After adjusting for individual-level, family-level, and PSU-level covariates, there are still significant random effects as follows: At the family level, $\rho_f = (1.068 + 0.121)/(1.068 + 0.121 + 3.29) = 0.265$, and at the PSU level, $\rho_p = 0.121/(1.068 + 0.121 + 3.29) = 0.027$.

Table 6.15 displays the regression coefficients for the fixed effects portion of the logistic model of neonatal mortality. Independent correlates of neonatal mortality include multiple births (AOR 9.72, 95% CI 8.97–10.5), birth intervals of less than 24 months (AOR 2.74, 95% CI 2.59–2.90), or 24–35 months (AOR 1.51, 95% CI 1.42–1.60), compared to longer intervals of 36 or more months, and first births (AOR 2.40, 95% CI 2.24–2.56). Elevated neonatal mortality also was independently associated with teenaged mothers (AOR 1.22, 95% CI 1.14–1.30), and older mothers: ages 30–34 years, OR 1.17, 95% CI 1.09–1.25, age 35 and above, AOR 1.31, 95% CI 1.19–1.44. Compared to Hindus,

Muslims had decreased neonatal mortality (AOR 0.83, 95% CI 0.77–0.88), as did Christians and those of other religions (AOR 0.70, 95% CI 0.64–0.76).

Babies born into scheduled tribe families had lower adjusted neonatal mortality (AOR 0.88, 95% CI 0.82–0.94). As standard of living increased, neonatal mortality declined; compared to the lowest asset index quintile, the adjusted odds ratio in the lower middle group was 0.91 (95% CI 0.86–0.96), and in the middle group it was 0.92 (95% CI 0.87–0.98). In the higher middle standard of living group the AOR was 0.84 (95% CI 0.79–0.90), and in the highest standard of living group, the adjusted odds ratio was 0.78 (95% CI 0.72–0.85). For both mothers and fathers, higher levels of education were independently associated with lower neonatal mortality. Compared to those with less educated mothers, having a mother educated through middle school improved the odds of survival through the neonatal period (AOR 0.88, 0.80–0.96), as did having a mother who completed high school (AOR 0.71, 95% CI 0.64–0.78). Babies of high school educated fathers had an adjusted odds ratio of 0.79 for neonatal mortality (95% CI 0.74–0.84), whereas those with middle school educated fathers had an AOR of 0.83 (95% CI 0.78–0.88).

Babies whose mothers were more mobile (i.e., moved to current location after the time of marriage) had poorer neonatal survival (AOR 1.14, 95% CI 1.09–1.20). Mother's media exposure was independently associated with a slightly decreased risk (AOR 0.97, 95% CI 0.94–1.00). Residing in the central and eastern regions of India conferred higher risk compared to South India, with adjusted odds ratios of 1.36 (95% CI 1.27–1.47) and 1.21 (95% CI 1.11–1.32), respectively. Also, residence in a location with a primary health center (AOR 0.87, 95% CI 0.81–0.94), or

Table 6.15. Neonatal mortality: Coefficient estimates from logistic regression model, main effects and interactions.

Fixed Effects	Coefficient	(SE)	AOR (95% CI)
Female Gender (vs. Male)	−0.337	(0.033)	(see interactions)
Year of Birth (vs. 1977–1983):			
1984–1989	−0.117	(0.049)	(see interactions)
1990–1999	−0.185	(0.050)	
Preceding Birth Interval (vs. 36+ Months):			
N/A (First Birth)	0.875	(0.034)	2.40 (2.24–2.56)
<24 Months	1.009	(0.029)	2.74 (2.59–2.90)
24–35 Months	0.410	(0.030)	1.51 (1.42–1.60)
Family Composition (vs. Birth Order 1 or 2):			
Birth Order 3/Surviving Older Brothers:			
None or One	−0.164	(0.040)	(see interactions)
Two	−0.356	(0.079)	
Birth Order 4+/Surviving Older Brothers:			
None or One	−0.163	(0.041)	
Two or More	−0.175	(0.043)	
Multiple Births	2.274	(0.041)	9.72 (8.97–10.5)

(continued)

Table 6.15. Neonatal mortality: Coefficient estimates from logistic regression model, main effects and interactions. *(continued)*

Fixed Effects	Coefficient	(SE)	AOR (95% CI)
Mother's Age at Time of Birth (vs. 25–29):			
<20	0.199	(0.033)	1.22 (1.14–1.30)
20–24	−0.021	(0.027)	0.98 (0.93–1.03)
30–34	0.155	(0.034)	1.17 (1.09–1.25)
35+	0.270	(0.049)	1.31 (1.19–1.44)
Propensity Score (vs. Q2 = 1.037–1.066):			
Q1 = SRB 0.898–1.037	−0.172	(0.064)	(see interactions)
Q3 = SRB 1.066–1.088	0.032	(0.054)	
Q4 = SRB 1.088–1.119	−0.063	(0.057)	
Q5 = SRB 1.119–1.364	0.026	(0.067)	
Religion (vs. Hindu):			
Muslim	−0.190	(0.034)	0.83 (0.77–0.88)
Christian/Other	−0.360	(0.043)	0.70 (0.64–0.76)
Scheduled Caste/Tribe (vs. Neither):			
Scheduled Caste	0.027	(0.026)	1.03 (0.98–1.08)
Scheduled Tribe	−0.130	(0.034)	0.88 (0.82–0.94)

	Coefficient	(SE)	
Household Standard of Living (vs. Low):			
Lower Middle	−0.098	(0.029)	0.91 (0.86–0.96)
Middle	−0.084	(0.030)	0.92 (0.87–0.98)
Higher Middle	−0.169	(0.033)	0.84 (0.79–0.90)
High	−0.246	(0.040)	0.78 (0.72–0.85)
Mother's Education (vs. < Middle School):			
Middle School	−0.129	(0.045)	0.88 (0.80–0.96)
High School+	−0.347	(0.047)	0.71 (0.64–0.78)
Father's Education (vs. Illiterate):			
< Middle School	−0.063	(0.024)	0.94 (0.90–0.98)
Middle School	−0.186	(0.032)	0.83 (0.78–0.88)
High School+	−0.238	(0.032)	0.79 (0.74–0.84)
Mother's Residence Before/After Marriage:			
Moved Here at Marriage (vs. Before)	−0.014	(0.023)	0.99 (0.94–1.03)
Moved Here After Marriage	0.135	(0.024)	1.14 (1.09–1.20)
Media Exposure	−0.030	(0.014)	0.97 (0.94–1.00)
Region (vs. Region 6: South):			
Region 1: North	−0.010	(0.046)	0.99 (0.90–1.08)
Region 2: West	−0.002	(0.045)	1.00 (0.91–1.09)
Region 3: Central	0.310	(0.037)	1.36 (1.27–1.47)
Region 4: East	0.192	(0.044)	1.21 (1.11–1.32)
Region 5: Northeast	−0.007	(0.048)	0.99 (0.90–1.09)

(continued)

Table 6.15. Neonatal mortality: Coefficient estimates from logistic regression model, main effects and interactions. *(continued)*

Fixed Effects	Coefficient	(SE)	AOR (95% CI)
Primary Health Center in Place of Residence	−0.137	(0.037)	0.87 (0.81–0.94)
Hospital in Place of Residence	−0.125	(0.042)	0.88 (0.81–0.96)
Urban Residence (vs. Rural)	0.061	(0.049)	1.06 (0.97–1.17)
Interactions			
*Gender * Family Composition:*			
Female * Birth Order 1–2	—	—	—
Female * Birth Order 3/0–1 Older Brothers	0.216	(0.055)	
Female * Birth Order 3/2 Older Brothers	0.093	(0.118)	
Female * Birth Order 4+/0–1 Older Brothers	0.323	(0.050)	
Female * Birth Order 4+/2+ Older Brothers	0.212	(0.051)	
*Year of Birth * Propensity Score:*			
1984–1989 * Q1 (Low)	0.209	(0.084)	—
1990–1999 * Q1 (Low)	0.184	(0.082)	
1984–1989 * Q3	−0.075	(0.072)	
1990–1999 * Q3	−0.139	(0.081)	

1984–1989 * Q4	0.001	(0.076)
1990–1999 * Q4	0.030	(0.077)
1984–1989 * Q5 (High)	−0.144	(0.084)
1990–1999 * Q5 (High)	−0.214	(0.087)
*Year of Birth * Gender * Propensity Score:*		
1984–1989 * Female * Q1 (Low)	0.029	(0.071)
1990–1999 * Female * Q1 (Low)	−0.070	(0.065)
1984–1989 * Female * Q3	0.178	(0.059)
1990–1999 * Female * Q3	−0.001	(0.081)
1984–1989 * Female * Q4	0.054	(0.068)
1990–1999 * Female * Q4	0.049	(0.068)
1984–1989 * Female * Q5 (High)	0.080	(0.073)
1990–1999 * Female * Q5 (High)	0.223	(0.077)

Random Effects	*Variance*	*(SE)*
Residual Variance Between PSUs (τ_{11})	0.121	(0.011)
Residual Variance Between Families (τ_{00})	1.068	(0.036)

a hospital (AOR 0.88, 95% CI 0.81–0.96) was independently associated with lower neonatal mortality. After controlling for the above factors, urban residence was no longer significantly associated with lower mortality (AOR 1.06, 95% CI 0.97–1.17).

Table 6.16 displays adjusted neonatal mortality odds ratios with 95% confidence intervals for those covariates with significant interaction terms. The effect of female gender on neonatal mortality varied according to the family composition of surviving older siblings. Female mortality was 71% of that of males (AOR 0.71, 95% CI 0.67–0.76) for first- and second-order births, but for third-order births, it depended upon the number of surviving older brothers: for those with one or fewer older brothers, the AOR was 0.88 (95% CI 0.80–0.98), but with two older brothers, the AOR was more favorable for girls at 0.78 (95% CI 0.62–0.98). Similarly, among fourth-order births, with one or fewer older brothers the neonatal survival of girls was no different than that of boys (AOR 0.98, 95% CI 0.89–1.08), but for fourth births with two or more surviving older brothers, neonatal mortality of girls was 88% of that of boys (AOR 0.88, 95% CI 0.80–0.97). The significant interaction between gender and family composition may also be interpreted as differing effects of family composition, depending upon the gender of the baby. For example, among boys, the risk is lower for third- and fourth-order births compared to first- and second-order births (AOR 0.70–0.85). However, among girls, the risk of neonatal mortality is elevated significantly for fourth-order births with one or fewer surviving older brothers (AOR 1.17, 95% CI 1.05–1.31) and is likely an indicator of female infanticide. A lower risk was found for the first-born girl in a family that already had two sons (AOR 0.77, 95% CI 0.59–1.00).

Table 6.16. Neonatal mortality odds ratios for variables with significant interactions.

Characteristic	AOR (95% CI)
*Family Composition * Gender (vs. Male):*	
Among Birth Order 1–2 * Female	0.71 (0.67–0.76)
Among Birth Order 3/0–1 Older Brothers * Female	0.88 (0.80–0.98)
Among Birth Order 3/2 Older Brothers * Female	0.78 (0.62–0.98)
Among Birth Order 4+/0–1 Older Brothers * Female	0.98 (0.89–1.08)
Among Birth Order 4+/2+ Older Brothers * Female	0.88 (0.80–0.97)
*Gender * Family Composition (vs. Birth Order 1–2):*	
Among Males:	
Birth Order 3/0–1 Older Brothers	0.85 (0.79–0.92)
Birth Order 3/2 Older Brothers	0.70 (0.60–0.82)
Birth Order 4+/0–1 Older Brothers	0.85 (0.78–0.92)
Birth Order 4+/2+ Older Brothers	0.84 (0.77–0.91)
Among Females:	
Birth Order 3/0–1 Older Brothers	1.05 (0.94–1.18)
Birth Order 3/2 Older Brothers	0.77 (0.59–1.00)
Birth Order 4+/0–1 Older Brothers	1.17 (1.05–1.31)
Birth Order 4+/2+ Older Brothers	1.04 (0.93–1.16)
*Propensity Score * Year of Birth (vs. 1977–1983):*	
Among Low SRB (Propensity Q1):	
1984–1989	1.09 (0.88–1.36)
1990–1999	1.00 (0.80–1.24)
Among Normal SRB (Propensity Q2):	
1984–1989	0.89 (0.81–0.97)
1990–1999	0.83 (0.75–0.91)
Among Slightly Elevated SRB (Propensity Q3):	
1984–1989	0.83 (0.68–1.01)
1990–1999	0.72 (0.58–0.90)
Among Moderately Elevated SRB (Propensity Q4):	
1984–1989	0.89 (0.72–1.09)
1990–1999	0.85 (0.69–1.05)

(continued)

Table 6.16. Neonatal mortality odds ratios for variables with significant interactions. *(continued)*

Characteristic	AOR (95% CI)
Among Highly Elevated SRB (Propensity Q5):	
1984–1989	0.77 (0.62–0.95)
1990–1999	0.67 (0.53–0.84)
*Propensity Score * Year of Birth * Gender (vs. Male):*	
Among Low SRB (Propensity Q1):	
1977–1983: Female	0.71 (0.67–0.76)
1984–1989: Female	0.74 (0.65–0.84)
1990–1999: Female	0.67 (0.59–0.75)
Among Normal SRB (Propensity Q2):	
1977–1983: Female	0.71 (0.67–0.76)
1984–1989: Female	0.71 (0.67–0.76)
1990–1999: Female	0.71 (0.67–0.76)
Among Slightly Elevated SRB (Propensity Q3):	
1977–1983: Female	0.71 (0.67–0.76)
1984–1989: Female	0.85 (0.77–0.95)
1990–1999: Female	0.71 (0.61–0.83)
Among Moderately Elevated SRB (Propensity Q4):	
1977–1983: Female	0.71 (0.67–0.76)
1984–1989: Female	0.75 (0.66–0.86)
1990–1999: Female	0.75 (0.66–0.85)
Among Highly Elevated SRB (Propensity Q5):	
1977–1983: Female	0.71 (0.67–0.76)
1984–1989: Female	0.77 (0.67–0.89)
1990–1999: Female	0.89 (0.77–1.03)

Interactions tested but found not to be statistically significant include gender by year of birth and gender by propensity quintile. There was an interaction between year of birth and propensity score quintile: Those in the higher quintiles experienced a greater decline in neonatal mortality over time. In the 5th propensity quintile (Q5), mortality in 1984–1989 was 77% of that in 1977–1983, and mortality in 1990–1999 was 67% of that in 1977–1983, while in Q1, there was no change over time, and in Q2 mortality dropped to 89% of its earlier level in 1984–1989 and to 83% in 1990–1999.

A significant and *positively* signed interaction was found for year of birth, female gender, and propensity score quintile. Over time, relative female neonatal mortality increased in the higher propensity quintiles. The neonatal mortality of girls was significantly lower than that of boys, with odds ratios ranging from 0.67 to 0.85, except in the highest propensity quintile in the 1990s, where the mortality of girls was 89% of that of boys and not significantly different than 1.0 (AOR 0.89, 95% CI 0.77–1.03). This odds ratio estimate increased over time in Q5 from a low of 0.71 in 1977–1983, to 0.77 in 1984–1989, and to 0.89 in 1990–1999. Q4 also saw a smaller increase in the relative mortality of girls over time: from 0.71 in 1977–1983 to 0.75 in 1984–1989 and remaining at 0.74 in 1990–1999.

These findings indicate that sex-selective abortion appears to not be substituting for neonatal mortality. Indeed, there is an additive effect whereby over time, female neonatal mortality has grown closer to male neonatal mortality among those most likely to practice sex selection of boys. Relative female neonatal survival has been deteriorating over time among those most likely to select for males.

Postneonatal Mortality

The family-level intraclass coefficient for the random intercept model with no covariates was: $\rho_f = (1.606 + 0.345)/(1.606 + 0.345 + 3.29) = 0.372$. Thus, 37% of the residual variance in postneonatal mortality is attributable to family, which is similar to that found for neonatal mortality. The residual variance attributable to Level 3 (PSU) is: ρ_p = 0.345/(1.606 + 0.345 + 3.29) = 0.066, which is slightly higher than that for neonatal mortality. The probability of postneonatal mortality in the unadjusted model is exp (–3.521)/[1 + exp (–3.521)] = 0.029, which is lower than the probability of neonatal mortality (0.044). After controlling for individual-level, family-level, and PSU-level covariates, there are still significant random effects as follows: at the family level, ρ_f = (0.863 + 0.156)/(0.863 + 0.156 + 3.29) = 0.236 and at the PSU level, ρ_p = 0.156/(0.863 + 0.156 + 3.29) = 0.036. Neonatal mortality had greater residual variance attributable to family (26.5%) than postneonatal mortality (23.6%), as would be expected due to the greater effect of genetic and biological factors on neonatal mortality. Postneonatal mortality had greater residual variance attributable to PSU (3.6%) than did neonatal mortality (2.7%) because of the importance of local services, such as immunizations and quality of health care. Table 6.17 displays logistic regression coefficients for the postneonatal mortality model, with odds ratios for fixed main effects. Higher risk of postneonatal mortality was found for multiple births (AOR 5.41, 95% CI 4.81–6.09), for shorter birth intervals of less than 24 months (AOR 2.65, 95% CI 2.48–2.84), for 24–35 months (AOR 1.56, 95% CI 1.46–1.68), and for first births (AOR 1.69, 95% CI 1.56–1.84). Postneonatal mortality was elevated for mothers under age 20 years (AOR 1.34, 95% CI 1.24–1.45), mothers aged 35 years and more (AOR 1.20, 95% CI 1.08–1.34), and lower for Muslims 0.77 (95% CI 0.71–0.83) and other religions 0.75 (95% CI 0.67–0.83) compared to Hindus. Risk of postneonatal mortality declined progressively as standard of living

Table 6.17. Postneonatal mortality: Coefficient estimates from logistic regression model, main effects and interactions.

Fixed Effects	Coefficient	(SE)	AOR (95% CI)
Female Gender (vs. Male)	−0.017	(0.052)	(see interactions)
Year of Birth (vs. 1977–1983):			
1984–1989	−0.198	(0.036)	(see interactions)
1990–1999	−0.388	(0.039)	
Preceding Birth Interval (vs. 36+ Months):			
N/A (First Birth)	0.525	(0.043)	1.69 (1.56–1.84)
<24 Months	0.975	(0.034)	2.65 (2.48–2.84)
24–35 Months	0.448	(0.036)	1.56 (1.46–1.68)
Family Composition (vs. Birth Order 1 or 2):			
Birth Order 3/Surviving Older Brothers:			(see interactions)
None or One	−0.075	(0.051)	
Two	0.052	(0.087)	
Birth Order 4+/Surviving Older Brothers:			
None or One	0.003	(0.051)	
Two or More	0.127	(0.052)	
Multiple Births	1.688	(0.060)	5.41 (4.81–6.09)

(continued)

Table 6.17. Postneonatal mortality: Coefficient estimates from logistic regression model, main effects and interactions. *(continued)*

Fixed Effects	Coefficient	(SE)	AOR (95% CI)
Mother's Age at Time of Birth (vs. 25–29):			
<20	0.291	(0.040)	1.34 (1.24–1.45)
20–24	0.075	(0.032)	1.08 (1.01–1.15)
30–34	0.039	(0.040)	1.04 (0.96–1.12)
35+	0.185	(0.055)	1.20 (1.08–1.34)
Propensity Score (vs. Q2 = 1.037–1.066):			
Q1 = SRB 0.898–1.037	−0.004	(0.049)	(see interactions)
Q3 = SRB 1.066–1.088	−0.111	(0.049)	
Q4 = SRB 1.088–1.119	−0.072	(0.050)	
Q5 = SRB 1.119–1.364	−0.214	(0.057)	
Religion (vs. Hindu):			
Muslim	−0.264	(0.041)	0.77 (0.96–0.83)
Christian/Other	−0.292	(0.052)	0.75 (0.67–0.83)
Scheduled Caste/Tribe (vs. Neither):			
Scheduled Caste	0.021	(0.031)	1.02 (0.96–1.09)
Scheduled Tribe	−0.066	(0.040)	0.94 (0.87–1.01)

Household Standard of Living (vs. Low):		
Lower Middle	−0.065 (0.033)	0.94 (0.88–1.00)
Middle	−0.192 (0.036)	0.83 (0.77–0.89)
Higher Middle	−0.228 (0.039)	0.80 (0.74–0.86)
High	−0.381 (0.050)	0.68 (0.62–0.75)
Mother's Education (vs. < Middle School):		
Middle School	−0.296 (0.062)	0.77 (0.66–0.84)
High School+	−0.528 (0.066)	0.59 (0.52–0.67)
Father's Education (vs. Illiterate):		
< Middle School	−0.070 (0.028)	0.93 (0.88–0.98)
Middle School	−0.151 (0.039)	0.86 (0.80–0.93)
High School+	−0.320 (0.039)	0.73 (0.67–0.78)
Mother's Labor Force Participation (vs. None):		
Noncash	0.010 (0.034)	1.01 (0.95–1.08)
Cash	0.059 (0.029)	1.06 (1.00–1.12)
Mother's Residence Before/After Marriage		
(vs. Lived in This Place Before Marriage):		
Moved Here at Marriage	−0.027 (0.027)	0.97 (0.92–1.03)
Moved Here After Marriage	0.146 (0.028)	1.16 (1.09–1.22)
Media Exposure	−0.061 (0.017)	0.94 (0.91–0.97)

(continued)

Table 6.17. Postneonatal mortality: Coefficient estimates from logistic regression model, main effects and interactions. *(continued)*

Fixed Effects	Coefficient	(SE)	AOR (95% CI)
Region (vs. Region 6: South):			
Region 1: North	0.371	(0.057)	1.45 (1.30–1.62)
Region 2: West	−0.041	(0.058)	0.96 (0.86–1.08)
Region 3: Central	0.507	(0.047)	1.66 (1.51–1.82)
Region 4: East	0.409	(0.054)	1.51 (1.35–1.67)
Region 5: Northeast	0.166	(0.059)	1.18 (1.05–1.33)
Primary Health Center in Place of Residence	−0.138	(0.045)	0.87 (0.80–0.95)
Hospital in Place of Residence	−0.058	(0.049)	0.94 (0.86–1.04)
Urban Residence (vs. Rural)	0.059	(0.059)	1.06 (0.94–1.19)
Interactions			
*Gender * Family Composition:*			
Female * Birth Order 1–2	—	—	—
Female * Birth Order 3/0–1 Older Brothers	0.115	(0.067)	
Female * Birth Order 3/2 Older Brothers	−0.371	(0.133)	
Female * Birth Order 4+/0–1 Older Brothers	0.290	(0.060)	
Female * Birth Order 4+/2 + Older Brothers	0.187	(0.059)	

*Gender * Propensity Score:*		
Female * Q1 (Low)	−0.114	(0.100)
Female * Q3	0.083	(0.089)
Female * Q4	0.086	(0.087)
Female * Q5 (High)	0.300	(0.101)
*Year of Birth * Gender * Propensity Score:*		
1984–1989 * Female * Q1 (Low)	0.054	(0.106)
1990–1999 * Female * Q1 (Low)	0.020	(0.099)
1984–1989 * Female * Q3	0.005	(0.086)
1990–1999 * Female * Q3	0.035	(0.098)
1984–1989 * Female * Q4	−0.018	(0.087)
1990–1999 * Female * Q4	−0.086	(0.093)
1984–1989 * Female * Q5 (High)	−0.185	(0.101)
1990–1999 * Female * Q5 (High)	−0.134	(0.108)
Random Effects	*Variance*	*(SE)*
Residual Variance Between PSU's (τ_{11})	0.156	(0.016)
Residual Variance Between Families (τ_{00})	0.863	(0.048)

increased. Those in the middle standard of living group had an AOR of 0.83 (95% CI 0.77–0.89), those in the higher middle group had an AOR of 0.80 (95% CI 0.74–0.86), whereas those in the highest standard of living group had a greatly reduced risk (AOR 0.68, 95% CI 0.62–0.75) compared to those in the lowest standard of living group.

Mother's education had a large impact on risk of postneonatal mortality. Infants with middle-school-educated mothers had 74% the risk of those whose mothers had less education (AOR 0.74, 95% CI 0.66–0.84), whereas children of high-school-educated mothers had 59% the risk (AOR 0.59, 95% CI 0.52–0.67). Father's education did not have as great an impact on postneonatal mortality as mother's level of education. Infants of middle-school-educated fathers had lower risk than infants of illiterate fathers (AOR 0.93, 95% CI 0.88–0.98), more so among infants of middle-school-educated (AOR 0.86, 95% CI 0.80–0.93), and high-school-educated fathers (AOR 0.73, 95% CI 0.67–0.78). Infants of mothers working for cash had slightly higher postneonatal mortality (AOR 1.06, 95% CI 1.00–1.12) compared to nonworking mothers; however, infants of unpaid working mothers did not (AOR 1.01, 95% CI 0.95–1.08). Infants of mothers who moved to their current location at some point after marriage had elevated risk (AOR 1.16, 95% CI 1.09–1.22), and mother's exposure to media lowered the risk (AOR 0.94, 95% CI 0.91–0.97). By region, only the Western states did not have higher risk than that in the Southern states. The highest risk was found in the Central states (AOR 1.66, 95% CI 1.51–1.82), the Eastern states (AOR 1.51, 95% CI 1.35–1.67), and the Northern states (AOR 1.45, 95% CI 1.30–1.62). The presence of a primary health center was associated with decreased risk (AOR 0.87,

95% CI 0.80–0.95) but not with the presence of a hospital (AOR 0.94, 95% CI 0.86–1.04).

Adjusted odds ratios with 95% confidence intervals are shown in Table 6.18 for those covariates with significant interaction terms. The gender differential in postneonatal mortality differed according to family composition.

Table 6.18. Postneonatal mortality odds ratios for variables with significant interactions.

Characteristic	AOR (95% CI)
*Family Composition * Gender (vs. Male):*	
Among Birth Order 1–2 * Female	0.98 (0.89–1.09)
Among Birth Order 3/0–1 Older Brothers * Female	1.10 (0.96–1.27)
Among Birth Order 3/2 Older Brothers * Female	1.31 (1.15–1.50)
Among Birth Order 4+/0–1 Older Brothers * Female	0.68 (0.52–0.88)
Among Birth Order 4+/2+ Older Brothers * Female	1.19 (1.05–1.34)
*Gender * Family Composition (vs. Birth Order 1–2):*	
Among Males:	
Birth Order 3/0–1 Older Brothers	0.93 (0.84–1.03)
Birth Order 3/2 Older Brothers	1.05 (0.89–1.25)
Birth Order 4+/0–1 Older Brothers	1.00 (0.91–1.11)
Birth Order 4+/2+ Older Brothers	1.14 (1.03–1.26)
Among Females:	
Birth Order 3/0–1 Older Brothers	1.04 (0.94–1.15)
Birth Order 3/2 Older Brothers	0.73 (0.59–0.89)
Birth Order 4+/0–1 Older Brothers	1.34 (1.22–1.48)
Birth Order 4+/2+ Older Brothers	1.37 (1.24–1.51)
*Propensity Score * Gender (vs. Male):*	
Among Low SRB (Q1) * Female	0.88 (0.73–1.05)
Among Normal SRB (Q2) * Female	0.98 (0.89–1.09)
Among Slightly Elevated SRB (Q3) * Female	1.07 (0.91–1.25)
Among Moderately Elevated SRB (Q4) * Female	1.07 (0.92–1.25)
Among Highly Elevated SRB (Q5) * Female	1.33 (1.11–1.59)

(continued)

Table 6.18. Postneonatal mortality odds ratios for variables with significant interactions. *(continued)*

Characteristic	AOR (95% CI)
*Propensity Score * Year of Birth * Gender (vs. Male):*	
Among Low SRB (Propensity Q1):	
1977–1983 * Female	0.88 (0.73–1.05)
1984–1989 * Female	0.93 (0.80–1.08)
1990–1999 * Female	0.90 (0.78–1.03)
Among Normal SRB (Propensity Q2):	
1977–1983 * Female	0.98 (0.89–1.09)
1984–1989 * Female	0.98 (0.89–1.09)
1990–1999 * Female	0.98 (0.89–1.09)
Among Slightly Elevated SRB (Propensity Q3):	
1977–1983 * Female	1.07 (0.91–1.25)
1984–1989 * Female	1.07 (0.90–1.28)
1990–1999 * Female	1.11 (0.90–1.36)
Among Moderately Elevated SRB (Propensity Q4):	
1977–1983 * Female	1.07 (0.92–1.25)
1984–1989 * Female	1.05 (0.88–1.26)
1990–1999 * Female	0.98 (0.81–1.19)
Among Highly Elevated SRB (Propensity Q5):	
1977–1983 * Female	1.33 (1.11–1.59)
1984–1989 * Female	1.10 (0.91–1.34)
1990–1999 * Female	1.16 (0.94–1.43)

Female infants were not at increased risk compared to boys if they were first or second born (AOR 0.98, 95% CI 0.89–1.09). They were not at significantly increased risk if they were third born with only one or no older brothers (AOR 1.10, 95% CI 0.96–1.27). They were at much lower risk than boys if they were third born and had two surviving older brothers (AOR 0.68, 95% CI 0.52–0.88), but fourth born girls were at elevated risk, even if they had two or more older brothers (AOR 1.19,

95% CI 1.05–1.34), and especially if they had no or only one older brother (AOR 1.31, 95% CI 1.15–1.50). The gender differential also increased with the propensity quintile: Girls in Q1 had an AOR of 0.88 (95% CI 0.73–1.05) compared to boys, Q2 an AOR of 0.98 (95% CI 0.89–1.09), Q3 an AOR of 1.07 (95% CI 0.91–1.25). Similarly, those in Q4 had an AOR of 1.07 (95% CI 0.92–1.25), and girls in Q5 had a significantly elevated AOR of 1.33 (95% CI 1.11–1.59). The interactions between gender and year of birth and between year of birth and propensity quintile were not found to be statistically significant. The three-way interaction terms between year of birth, female gender, and propensity score quintile were not statistically significant but were included in the model, and gender differential point estimates with 95% confidence intervals were calculated for descriptive purposes. The AOR for girls relative to boys increased as the propensity increased with no change over time for quintiles 1 through 3: The AOR in Q1 ranged from 0.88–0.93 over the three time periods and did not differ statistically from 1.00; Q2 was the reference category with an AOR estimate of 0.98 for the three time periods; in Q3 the AOR ranged from 1.07–1.11 over time; in Q4 the AOR for girls declined over time from 1.07 to 1.05 in the 1980s, to 0.98 in the 1990s; and in the highest propensity quintile, girls had significantly elevated postneonatal mortality in the early time period (AOR 1.33, 95% CI 1.11–1.59), with a decline over time to 1.10 in the mid- to late 1980s, and to 1.16 in the 1990s. This trend in the upper propensity quintiles suggests that there is some substitution of sex-selective abortion for postneonatal mortality occurring, but the confidence intervals are wide, with a great degree of overlap, so definitive inferences cannot be made.

Child Mortality

The family-level intraclass coefficient for the random intercept model of child mortality with no covariates was: $\rho_f = (1.865 + 0.559)/(1.865 + 0.345 + 3.29) = 0.424$. Thus, 42% of the residual variance in child mortality is attributable to family before adjustment for covariates. The residual variance in child mortality attributable to Level 3 (PSU) is: $\rho_p = 0.559/(1.865 + 0.559 + 3.29) = 0.098$, which is higher than that for either neonatal or postneonatal mortality. The probability of a 12-month-old child not surviving to the age of 5 years in the unadjusted model is $\exp(-3.678)/[1 + \exp(-3.678)] = 0.025$, which is slightly lower than the probability of postneonatal mortality (0.029). After controlling for individual-level, family-level, and PSU-level covariates, there are still significant random effects as follows: at the family level, $\rho_f = (0.613 + 0.205)/(0.613 + 0.205 + 3.29) = 0.199$, and at the PSU level, $\rho_p = 0.205/(0.613 + 0.205 + 3.29) = 0.050$. After adjustment for covariates, there is less residual variance attributable to family (19.9%) for child mortality than for either postneonatal mortality (23.6%) or neonatal mortality (26.5%) because child survival is more dependent upon social factors. This is also reflected in the greater residual variance attributable to PSU (5%) for child mortality than postneonatal (3.6%) or neonatal (2.7%) mortality.

Independent risk factors for child mortality identified in the multivariate model are shown in Table 6.19. Shorter preceding birth intervals of <24 months (AOR 2.29, 95% CI 2.13–2.47), or 24–35 months (AOR 1.63, 95% CI 1.51–1.75) were associated with increased risk. Shorter subsequent birth intervals of <24 months (AOR 1.71, 95% CI 1.60–1.82) or 24–35 months (AOR 1.08, 95% CI 1.01–1.16) were also associated with higher risk of child mortality. Multiple births surviving to the age of 1 year had double the risk of not surviving to age 5 as singleton births (AOR 2.06, 95% CI 1.70–2.50). Children of young mothers <20 years of age had an elevated risk (AOR 1.22, 95% CI 1.14–1.30), as did children of older mothers 30–34 years of age (AOR 1.17, 95% CI 1.09–1.25), and especially those with mothers aged 35 and older (AOR 1.31, 95% CI 1.19–1.44).

Children in non-Hindu families had 80% the risk of those in Hindu families: The adjusted odds ratio for Muslims was 0.81 (95% CI 0.75–0.89), and for Christian and other religions it was 0.80 (95% CI 0.71–0.89). Children of schedule castes (AOR 1.12, 95% CI 1.05–1.19) and scheduled tribes (AOR 1.13, 95% CI 1.04–1.22) had a similar level of elevated risk. The gradient by standard of living was sharper than for neonatal or postneonatal mortality, with odds ratios declining from 0.87 in the lower middle group to 0.74 in the middle group, to 0.59 in the higher middle group, and finally to 0.54 in the highest standard of living group. The gradient by mother's and father's educational level was similarly steep: Children of middle-school-educated mothers had an adjusted odds ratio of 0.56 (95% CI 0.47–0.66) compared to children of less educated mothers, and children of high-school-educated mothers had an adjusted odds ratio of 0.47 (95% CI 0.39–0.56). Children of middle-school-educated fathers had an AOR of 0.74 (95% CI 0.68–0.81), whereas those with a high-school-educated father had an AOR of 0.64 (95% CI 0.59–0.70).

Children of working mothers had poorer survival than those of nonworking mothers; noncash workers had a 14% increase in risk (AOR 1.14, 95% CI 1.06–1.22) and cash workers had a 23% increase in risk (AOR 1.23, 95% CI 1.16–1.31). Children

Table 6.19. Child mortality: Coefficient estimates from logistic regression model, main effects and interactions.

Fixed Effects	Coefficient	(SE)	AOR (95% CI)
Female Gender (vs. Male)	0.258	(0.046)	(see interactions)
Year of Birth (vs. 1977–1983):			(see interactions)
1984–1989	−0.206	(0.062)	
1990–1999	−0.356	(0.070)	
Preceding Birth Interval (vs. 36+ Months):			
N/A (First Birth)	0.219	(0.048)	1.24 (1.13–1.37)
<24 Months	0.830	(0.037)	2.29 (2.13–2.47)
24–35 Months	0.486	(0.037)	1.63 (1.51–1.75)
Subsequent Birth Interval (vs. 36+ Months):			
N/A (Last Birth)	−0.632	(0.040)	0.53 (0.49–0.57)
<24 Months	0.537	(0.033)	1.71 (1.60–1.82)
24–35 Months	0.078	(0.035)	1.08 (1.01–1.16)
Family Composition (vs. Birth Order 1 or 2): *Birth Order 3/Surviving Older Brothers:*			(see interactions)
None or One	0.053	(0.057)	
Two	0.290	(0.094)	

Birth Order 4+/Surviving Older Brothers:			
None or One	0.041	(0.059)	
Two or More	0.434	(0.056)	2.06 (1.70–2.50)
Multiple Births	0.724	(0.098)	
Mother's Age at Time of Birth (vs. 25–29):			
<20	0.209	(0.044)	1.22 (1.14–1.30)
20–24	0.076	(0.034)	0.98 (0.93–1.03)
30–34	0.044	(0.043)	1.17 (1.09–1.25)
35+	0.164	(0.061)	1.31 (1.19–1.44)
Propensity Score (vs. Q2 = 1.037–1.066):			
Q1 = SRB 0.898–1.037	−0.017	(0.076)	(see interactions)
Q3 = SRB 1.066–1.088	0.034	(0.067)	
Q4 = SRB 1.088–1.119	0.037	(0.070)	
Q5 = SRB 1.119–1.364	0.175	(0.084)	
Religion (vs. Hindu):			
Muslim	−0.206	(0.045)	0.81 (0.75–0.89)
Christian/Other	−0.226	(0.058)	0.80 (0.71–0.89)
Scheduled Caste/Tribe (vs. Neither):			
Scheduled Caste	0.112	(0.033)	1.12 (1.05–1.19)
Scheduled Tribe	0.120	(0.041)	1.13 (1.04–1.22)

(continued)

Table 6.19. Child mortality: Coefficient estimates from logistic regression model, main effects and interactions. *(continued)*

Fixed Effects	Coefficient	(SE)	AOR (95% CI)
Household Standard of Living (vs. Low):			
Lower Middle	-0.134	(0.034)	0.87 (0.82–0.93)
Middle	-0.296	(0.037)	0.74 (0.69–0.80)
Higher Middle	-0.526	(0.044)	0.59 (0.54–0.64)
High	-0.610	(0.057)	0.54 (0.49–0.61)
Mother's Education (vs. < Middle School):			
Middle School	-0.585	(0.083)	0.56 (0.47–0.66)
High School+	-0.764	(0.094)	0.47 (0.39–0.56)
Father's Education (vs. Illiterate):			
<Middle School	-0.159	(0.030)	0.85 (0.80–0.90)
Middle School	-0.295	(0.044)	0.74 (0.68–0.81)
High School+	-0.439	(0.044)	0.64 (0.59–0.70)
Mother's Labor Force Participation (vs. None):			
Noncash	0.127	(0.036)	1.14 (1.06–1.22)
Cash	0.207	(0.031)	1.23 (1.16–1.31)
Mother's Residence Before/After Marriage *(vs. Lived in This Place Before Marriage):*			
Moved Here at Marriage	-0.055	(0.030)	0.95 (0.89–1.00)
Moved Here after Marriage	0.104	(0.031)	1.11 (1.04–1.18)

Media Exposure	−0.072	(0.019)	0.93 (0.90–0.97)
Region (vs. Region 6: South):			
Region 1: North	0.001	(0.066)	1.00 (0.88–1.14)
Region 2: West	−0.016	(0.064)	0.98 (0.87–1.12)
Region 3: Central	0.540	(0.052)	1.72 (1.55–1.90)
Region 4: East	0.007	(0.064)	1.01 (0.89–1.14)
Region 5: Northeast	0.061	(0.066)	1.06 (0.93–1.21)
Primary Health Center in Place of Residence	−0.029	(0.048)	0.97 (0.88–1.07)
Hospital in Place of Residence	−0.122	(0.054)	0.89 (0.80–0.98)
Urban Residence (vs. Rural)	0.016	(0.066)	1.02 (0.89–1.16)
Interactions			
*Gender * Family Composition (vs. Male):*			
Female * Birth Order 1–2	—	—	—
Female * Birth Order 3/0–1 Older Brothers	0.163	(0.071)	
Female * Birth Order 3/2 Older Brothers	0.048	(0.125)	
Female * Birth Order 4+/0–1 Older Brothers	0.324	(0.068)	
Female * Birth Order 4+/2+ Older Brothers	0.011	(0.063)	
*Year of Birth * Propensity Score:*			
1984–1989 * Q1 (Low)	0.129	(0.112)	
1990–1999 * Q1 (Low)	0.010	(0.110)	
1984–1989 * Q3	0.044	(0.093)	

(continued)

Table 6.19. Child mortality: Coefficient estimates from logistic regression model, main effects and interactions. *(continued)*

Fixed Effects	Coefficient	(SE)	AOR (95% CI)
1990–1999 * Q3	-0.164	(0.119)	—
1984–1989 * Q4	0.110	(0.097)	
1990–1999 * Q4	-0.234	(0.119)	
1984–1989 * Q5 (High)	0.002	(0.110)	
1990–1999 * Q5 (High)	-0.335	(0.136)	
*Year of Birth * Gender * Propensity Score:*			
1984–1989 * Female * Q1 (Low)	-0.173	(0.102)	—
1990–1999 * Female * Q1 (Low)	-0.184	(0.090)	
1984–1989 * Female * Q3	0.004	(0.075)	
1990–1999 * Female * Q3	0.202	(0.113)	
1984–1989 * Female * Q4	-0.031	(0.081)	
1990–1999 * Female * Q4	0.081	(0.113)	
1984–1989 * Female * Q5 (High)	-0.075	(0.089)	
1990—1999 * Female * Q5 (High)	0.040	(0.131)	

Random Effects	Variance	SE	
Residual Variance Between PSUs (τ_{11})	0.205	(0.019)	—
Residual Variance Between Families (τ_{00})	0.613	(0.047)	—

of mothers who were more mobile had an elevated odds ratio of 1.11 (95% CI 1.04–1.18) compared to mothers who lived in their current place of residence prior to marriage. Media exposure of mothers had an independent protective effect on child mortality (AOR 0.93, 95% CI 0.90–0.97).

Children residing in the states of Central India had significantly elevated mortality compared to the Southern states (AOR 1.72, 95% CI 1.55–1.90). The presence of a primary health center did not significantly lower the mortality risk (AOR 0.97, 95% CI 0.88–1.07), but the presence of a hospital did (AOR 0.89, 95% CI 0.80–0.98). The urban/rural mortality differential vanished after controlling for these other factors (AOR 1.02, 95% CI 0.89–1.16).

Table 6.20 displays adjusted odds ratios calculated from the significant interaction terms in the logistic regression model. As was the case for infant mortality, the magnitude of the gender differential in child mortality depended upon the family composition of surviving siblings. Higher order births with one or fewer surviving older brother had the greatest gender differential in child mortality: Girls born fourth and higher with zero or one surviving older brothers had 79% higher risk of mortality than similarly situated boys (AOR 1.79, 95% CI 1.58–2.03), whereas among third-born children with zero or one older brothers, girls had 52% higher risk than boys (AOR 1.52, 95% CI 1.34–1.74). The adjusted odds ratios for girls were significantly elevated, but to a lesser degree, for each of the other family composition categories: first- or second-order births (AOR 1.29, 95% CI 1.18–1.42), third-order births with 2 older brothers (AOR 1.36, 95% CI 1.07–1.73), and fourth- and higher order births with at least two older brothers (AOR 1.28, 95% CI 1.14–1.43). Among boys, those with at least two older brothers had a higher risk of child mortality. Third-born boys with two older brothers had an adjusted odds ratio of 1.34 (95% CI 1.11–1.61) versus first- and second-born boys, and boys who were fourth- and higher order births with at least two surviving older brothers had an even higher adjusted odds ratio of 1.54 (95% CI 1.38–1.72).

Table 6.20. Child mortality odds ratios for variables with significant interactions.

Characteristic	AOR (95% CI)
*Family Composition * Gender (vs. Male):*	
Among Birth Order 1–2 * Female	1.29 (1.18–1.42)
Among Birth Order 3/0–1 Older Brothers * Female	1.52 (1.34–1.74)
Among Birth Order 3/2 Older Brothers * Female	1.36 (1.07–1.73)
Among Birth Order 4+/0–1 Older Brothers * Female	1.79 (1.58–2.03)
Among Birth Order 4+/2+ Older Brothers * Female	1.28 (1.14–1.43)
*Gender * Family Composition (vs. Birth Order 1–2):*	
Among Males:	
Birth Order 3/0–1 Older Brothers	1.05 (0.94–1.18)
Birth Order 3/2 Older Brothers	1.34 (1.11–1.61)
Birth Order 4+/0–1 Older Brothers	1.04 (0.93–1.17)
Birth Order 4+/2+ Older Brothers	1.54 (1.38–1.72)
Among Females:	
Birth Order 3/0–1 Older Brothers	1.24 (1.07–1.44)
Birth Order 3/2 Older Brothers	1.40 (1.05–1.87)
Birth Order 4+/0–1 Older Brothers	1.44 (1.25–1.66)
Birth Order 4+/2+ Older Brothers	1.53 (1.34–1.74)
*Propensity Score * Year of Birth (vs. 1977–1983):*	
Among Low SRB (Propensity Q1):	
1984–1989	0.93 (0.77–1.11)
1990–1999	0.71 (0.59–0.84)

(continued)

Table 6.20. Child mortality odds ratios for variables with significant interactions. *(continued)*

Characteristic	AOR (95% CI)
Among Normal SRB (Propensity Q2):	
1984–1989	0.81 (0.72–0.92)
1990–1999	0.70 (0.61–0.80)
Among Slightly Elevated SRB (Propensity Q3):	
1984–1989	0.85 (0.74–0.98)
1990–1999	0.59 (0.49–0.72)
Among Moderately Elevated SRB (Propensity Q4):	
1984–1989	0.91 (0.79–1.05)
1990–1999 – Q4	0.55 (0.46–0.67)
Among Highly Elevated SRB (Propensity Q5):	
1984–1989	0.82 (0.68–0.97)
1990–1999	0.50 (0.40–0.63)
*Propensity Score * Year of Birth * Gender*	
(vs. Male):	
Among Low SRB (Propensity Q1):	
1977–1983 * Female	1.29 (1.18–1.42)
1984–1989 * Female	1.09 (0.90–1.32)
1990–1999 * Female	1.08 (0.90–1.28)
Among Normal SRB (Propensity Q2):	
1977–1983 * Female	1.29 (1.18–1.42)
1984–1989 * Female	1.29 (1.18–1.42)
1990–1999 * Female	1.29 (1.18–1.42)
Among Slightly Elevated SRB (Propensity Q3):	
1977–1983 * Female	1.29 (1.18–1.42)
1984–1989 * Female	1.30 (1.13–1.49)
1990–1999 * Female	1.58 (1.27–1.97)
Among Moderately Elevated SRB (Propensity Q4):	
1977–1983 * Female	1.29 (1.18–1.42)
1984–1989 * Female	1.26 (1.08–1.46)
1990–1999 * Female	1.40 (1.13–1.74)
Among Highly Elevated SRB (Propensity Q5):	
1977–1983 * Female	1.29 (1.18–1.42)
1984–1989 * Female	1.20 (1.01–1.44)
1990–1999 * Female	1.35 (1.05–1.74)

The degree of decline over time in child mortality varied by the propensity score quintile. Although children in all propensity quintiles experienced a progressive decline over time in mortality, the greatest drop was found among those in the highest propensity score quintiles. Those in Q5 had the largest relative decrease, with an AOR of 0.82 in 1984–1989 compared to the earliest time period of 1977–1983, declining to 0.50 in 1990–1999. Those in Q4 had adjusted odds ratios of 0.91 and 0.55, in 1984–1989 and 1990–1999, respectively, and in Q3 the adjusted odds ratios declined to 0.85 and 0.59 over time. The decline over time in child mortality was less extensive in the lower propensity score quintiles: Among those in Q2, the adjusted odds ratio was 0.81 in 1984–1989, and 0.70 in 1990–1999, and among those in the lowest propensity quintile the AORs declined from 0.93 to 0.71 over time.

The gender differential, on the other hand, exhibited a very different pattern over time, declining significantly only in the lowest propensity score quintile. Girls were 29% more likely to die by the age of 5 years than boys in the earliest time period (AOR 1.29, 95% CI 1.18–1.42). That differential declined in the mid- to late-1980s among those in Q1 to 9% (AOR 1.09, 95% CI 0.90–1.32) and stayed at that level in the 1990s (AOR 1.08, 95% CI 0.90–1.28). There were no significant changes in the gender differential over time in the other propensity score quintiles. The point estimates decreased in the 1984–1989 period and then increased to a higher level in the 1990s in the two upper quintiles. Among those in Q4, the AOR declined from 1.29 in 1977–1983 to 1.26 in 1984–1989 and then increased to 1.40 in the 1990s. Similarly, among those in Q5 the AOR for girls relative to boys initially declined from 1.29 to 1.20 in 1984–1989 and then increased to 1.35 in 1990–1999. Thus, there is no evidence that sex-selective abortion is substituting for child mortality.

SUMMARY OF FINDINGS

The contingency table analysis, the AUC analysis, and the multivariate analysis all indicate that there has been an additive effect of sex-selective abortion on neonatal mortality. Rather than female mortality improving among those most likely to sex select for males, it has been deteriorating over time, to the point where the biological advantage that females have in the neonatal period has largely disappeared.

The AUC analysis and the multivariate analysis of postneonatal mortality both indicate that sex-selective abortion has not had an impact upon excess female mortality in the postneonatal period. The multivariate interactions showed a trend toward a narrowing gender differential over time among those with the highest propensity for sex selection, but the interaction terms were not statistically significant.

The AUC analysis of child mortality showed a slight decline in the absolute gender differential in the 1990s among those most likely to utilize sex-selective abortion. The multivariate analysis showed no significant effects of sex-selective abortion on child mortality. There was, however, a nonsignificant initial decline in relative female child mortality in the mid- to late-1980s, but that trend was reversed in the 1990s.

CHAPTER 7

THE EFFECT OF
PRENATAL SEX SELECTION
ON GENDER DIFFERENTIALS
IN HEALTH CARE
AND MORBIDITY

Gender differentials in children's preventive and curative health care and child morbidity were examined in the analysis presented in this chapter. Data on care and morbidity were available only for surviving children under the age of 3 years at the time of the survey; thus, changes in gender disparities could only be examined over the decade of the 1990s. The analyses were similar to those presented in the previous chapter on mortality. The research hypothesis being tested is whether those with the highest propensity for sex selection experienced lower gender differentials in health care and morbidity. Girls born into families that practice prenatal selection are more likely to be wanted than girls born into families not practicing prenatal selection; thus, it is hypothesized that they will have higher levels of health care and lower levels of morbidity than other girls and levels equivalent to boys born into similar families. This trend should become more pronounced over the decade of the 1990s, as sex-selective abortion has diffused. If the data support this hypothesis, then that would provide evidence of a pathway through which substitution might operate.

Preventive Care

Use of preventive care was measured as the proportion of children aged 12–23 months at the time of the survey who were fully vaccinated. Full vaccination included the following immunizations: BCG, measles, a series of three polio, and a series of three DPT injections. The outcome was framed in the negative as lack of full vaccination in order that an elevated odds ratio for girls would indicate a greater gender differential in preventive care. Data were combined for the two NFHS surveys, so the birth years included were 1990–1992 for NFHS-1 and 1996–1999 for NFHS-2.

Child-Level Characteristics

The majority of children aged 12–23 months in surveyed households were not fully immunized. Overall, 63% of children were not fully vaccinated. As shown in Table 7.1, this proportion varied by gender, year of birth, multiple births, age of the mother, birth order, family composition, and propensity score. Girls had higher rates of incomplete vaccination than boys; 64.2% of girls and 61.9% of boys were found to not have full vaccination (p = 0.01). Incomplete vaccination declined significantly over time from 66.6% in the early 1990s to 58.4% in the late 1990s (p < 0.001). A greater proportion of twins and triplets were not fully vaccinated (76.6%) compared to singleton births (62.8%) (p = 0.002). The rate of incomplete vaccination was lowest among children of mothers in their early 20s (58.7%), and it increased as the age of the mother increased to a maximum of 79.9% among children of mothers aged 35 and older (p < 0.001). The rate was slightly elevated among teenaged mothers, with 63.5% of children not fully vaccinated.

Lack of full immunization increased with increasing birth order, from 52.1% of first-born children to 77.8% of fourth- and higher order births (p < 0.001). Moreover, among third and higher births, having older brothers was associated with lower vaccination rates. Within each birth order, the incomplete vaccination rate increased with the number of surviving older brothers from 61.3% of third births with no older brothers to 66.8% of third-born children with two older brothers. Similarly, 70.8% of fourth-born children with no older brothers were lacking complete vaccination compared to 82.1% of forth-born children with two or more older brothers.

By propensity score, the best vaccination rates were found among the children in Q5, the highest propensity quintile, with 48.3% of children not completely vaccinated, and the worst vaccination rates were among children in the lowest propensity quintile (Q1), with 59.0% of children unvaccinated. In the three middle quintiles the rate did not vary much, ranging from 62% to 65%.

Table 7.1. Preventive care by child-level characteristics.

Characteristic	Number of Children	% Not Fully Vaccinated	p-value
Overall	19,780	63.0%	—
Gender:			
Male	10,263	61.9%	
Female	9,517	64.2%	0.01
Year of Birth:			
1990–1992 – NFHS-1	10,883	66.6%	
1996–1999 – NFHS-2	8,897	58.4%	<0.001
Multiple Births:			
No	19,512	62.8%	
Yes	268	76.6%	0.002
Mother's Age at Time of Birth:			
<20	4,083	63.5%	
20–24	7,508	58.7%	
25–29	4,982	62.6%	
30–34	2,189	70.6%	
35+	1,018	79.9%	<0.001

Birth Order:			
1	5,486	52.1%	
2	4,951	56.2%	
3	3,515	63.7%	
4+	5,828	77.8%	<0.001
Family Composition (Siblings):			
Birth Order 1	5,486	52.1%	<0.001
Birth Order 2:			
No surviving older brothers	2,629	57.7%	
One surviving older brother	2,322	54.6%	
Birth Order 3:			
No surviving older brothers	1,167	61.3%	
One surviving older brother	1,706	64.2%	
Two surviving older brothers	642	66.8%	
Birth Order 4 or Higher:			
No surviving older brothers	917	70.8%	
One surviving older brothers	2,106	75.0%	
Two or more surv older bros	2,805	82.1%	<0.001
Propensity Score (Quintiles):			
Q1 = SRB 0.898–1.037	5,185	69.0%	
Q2 = SRB 1.037–1.066	3,617	61.9%	
Q3 = SRB 1.066–1.088	2,895	63.4%	
Q4 = SRB 1.088–1.119	3,787	65.3%	
Q5 = SRB 1.119–1.364	4,129	48.3%	<0.001

Family-Level Characteristics

Muslim families had high rates of incomplete vaccination, with 72.4% of children unvaccinated, compared to 62.4% of Hindu children, 50.7% of Christian children, and 40.0% of children of other religions (p < 0.001), as shown in Table 7.2. Seventy-five percent of the children of scheduled tribe families were not vaccinated compared to 67% of scheduled caste children and 60.4% of other children (p < 0.001). The proportion of children not fully vaccinated declined precipitously as the level of family's standard of living increased. Seventy-five percent of those in the lowest standard of living category were unvaccinated compared to 66.0% of those in the middle and 39.3% of those in the highest standard of living categories (p < 0.001). Similar gradients were found by the mother's level of education, with 75% of children of illiterate mothers unvaccinated and 31% of children of high-school-educated mothers unvaccinated, and by the father's level of education, with 78% of children of illiterate fathers and 47% of children of high school graduates unvaccinated. Mothers who were employed but did not earn cash had a greater proportion of children who were not vaccinated (67.6%) compared to children of unemployed mothers (62.4%) and children of mothers who worked for cash (62.3%). There was a small decline in the proportion unvaccinated by the length of mother's residence in her present location; those who moved to the present location after marriage had the highest level of 64.5% unvaccinated compared to 64.0% of those who moved at the time of marriage and 61.1% of those who lived at their present location prior to marriage (p = 0.003).

Native speakers of Group 2 languages (Marathi and Konkani), representing the Southern Indo-Aryan cultural pattern, had the lowest proportion of unvaccinated children (30.7%), followed by native speakers of Group 4 languages (40.7%), which include the Southern languages of Telegu, Tamil, Kannada, and Malayalam, representing the Dravidian cultural pattern. Group 1 languages include Hindi, Bengali, Punjabi, Gujarati, Urdu, and Kashmiri and represent the core Aryan cultural pattern. Native speakers of these languages had the highest proportion of unvaccinated children (71.9%). A large percentage of unvaccinated children (68.6%) was found among speakers of other languages that include Assamese, Sindhi, English, and all other native tongues not falling into the first three groups.

The mother's level of media exposure was associated with vaccination of the children. Children of mothers who were not exposed to any media (radio, television, or cinema) had a high percentage of incomplete vaccination (76.7%) compared to mothers with one media source (56.2%) and two (40.8%) or three (39.1%) sources ($p < 0.001$).

PSU-Level Characteristics

Table 7.3 displays the percentages of children who are not fully vaccinated by PSU-level characteristics. Urban children were much more likely to receive full vaccination than rural children. Sixty-eight percent of rural children were not fully vaccinated, compared to 47.9% of urban children ($p < 0.001$). Lower rates of incomplete vaccination were found in the Western region (37.7%), the Northern region (40.6%), and the Southern region (41.6%), and high rates were found in the Central region (81.6%), the Northeast (79.9%), and a moderate rate in the East region (61.6%).

The presence of a primary health center in the village was associated with a lower percentage of incomplete vaccination

Table 7.2. Preventive care by family-level characteristics.

Characteristic	Number of Children	% Not Fully Vaccinated	p-value
Religion:			
Hindu	14,835	62.4%	
Muslim	2,744	72.4%	
Christian	1,283	50.7%	
Other	909	40.0%	<0.001
Scheduled Caste/Tribe:			
Scheduled Caste	3,077	67.0%	
Scheduled Tribe	2,781	75.0%	
Neither	13,843	60.4%	<0.001
Household Standard of Living (Quintiles):			
Low	3,858	75.1%	
Lower Middle	3,907	72.8%	
Middle	3,940	66.0%	
Higher Middle	4,068	56.7%	
High	4,007	39.3%	<0.001
Mother's Education:			
Illiterate	11,516	75.1%	
< Middle School	3,547	51.3%	
Middle School	1,851	40.3%	
High School+	2,865	31.1%	<0.001

Father's Education:			
Illiterate	6,024	78.1%	
< Middle School	5,074	63.3%	
Middle School	2,840	55.9%	
High School+	5,751	47.4%	<0.001
Mother's Labor Force Participation:			
None	13,677	62.4%	
Noncash	2,581	67.6%	
Cash	3,510	62.3%	0.002
Mother's Residence Here Before/After Marriage:			
Lived Here Before Marriage	7,848	61.1%	
Moved Here at Marriage	7,647	64.0%	
Moved Here After Marriage	4,285	64.6%	0.003
Mother Tongue:			
Group 1	11,694	71.9%	
Group 2	1,061	30.7%	
Group 4	2,740	40.7%	
Other	4,278	68.6%	<0.001
Media Exposure:			
None	9,255	76.7%	
One	5,419	56.2%	
Two	4,139	40.8%	
Three	967	39.1%	<0.001

Table 7.3. Preventive care by PSU-level characteristics.

Characteristic	Number of Children	% Not Fully Vaccinated	p-value
Urban/Rural Residence:			
Urban	5,346	47.9%	
Rural	14,434	67.5%	<0.001
Region:			
Region 1: North	3,157	40.6%	
Region 2: West	2,092	37.7%	
Region 3: Central	7,353	81.6%	
Region 4: East	1,769	61.6%	
Region 5: Northeast	2,486	79.9%	
Region 6: South	2,923	41.6%	<0.001
Primary Health Center in Village:			
No	12,088	68.7%	
Yes	1,941	58.0%	<0.001
Mobile Health Unit in Village:			
No	11,571	67.0%	
Yes	2,650	68.3%	0.46

Clinic in Village:			
No	9,579	68.8%	
Yes	3,664	61.1%	<0.001
Nearest Hospital to Village (Quintiles):			
0–3 km	3,108	60.1%	
4–7 km	2,858	65.1%	
8–12 km	2,850	68.5%	
13–21 km	2,383	70.6%	
≥22 km	2,852	73.2%	<0.001
Nearest Town to Village (Quintiles):			
0–5 km	2,996	64.7%	
6–9 km	2,502	66.9%	
10–14 km	2,689	63.9%	
15–24 km	2,978	67.6%	
≥25 km	3,112	72.6%	<0.001
Electricity in Village:			
No	2,664	84.6%	
Yes	11,563	62.5%	<0.001

(continued)

Table 7.3. Preventive care by PSU-level characteristics. *(continued)*

Characteristic	Number of Children	% Not Fully Vaccinated	p-value
Television in Village:			
No	2,081	81.5%	
Yes	11,927	65.0%	<0.001
Number of Households in Village (Quintiles):			
<125	2,753	72.0%	
125–248	2,759	70.6%	
249–400	2,787	70.0%	
401–744	2,496	66.8%	
745–8,930	2,760	56.0%	<0.001

(58.0%), as was the presence of a clinic (61.1%). There was a gradient of increasing percentage of unvaccinated children as the distance to the nearest hospital increased from 60% among those closest to a hospital to 73% among those furthest from a hospital. The presence of a mobile health unit in the village was not associated with the rate of vaccination. A higher proportion of children were unvaccinated if they lived 25 or more kilometers from a town (72.6%) versus those living closer (64–68%). Villages with electricity, television, and a greater number of households had a greater percentage of vaccinated children. Sixty-two percent of children were not vaccinated in villages with electricity, compared to 85% of those living in villages without electricity. Similarly, children living in villages without any televisions had a high rate of incomplete vaccination (81.5%) versus those living in a village with at least one television (65.0%). By the number of households in the village, there was a gradient from 56% of children unvaccinated among villages with the highest number of households to 72% unvaccinated among villages with the fewest number of households.

Gender Differential by Propensity Score and Year of Birth

Table 7.4 displays a contingency table analysis of the gender differential in preventive care by year of birth and propensity score quintile. In the early 1990s, girls were 12% more likely to be unvaccinated than boys (OR 1.12, 95% CI 1.02–1.24), decreasing slightly to 9% by the late 1990s (OR 1.09, 95% CI 0.98–1.21). When stratified by propensity score quintile, the gender differential decreased over time in every quintile except the 1st and the 5th, Q1 and Q5. In the lowest propensity quintile,

Table 7.4. Preventive care by year of birth, propensity score quintile, and gender, India, 1990–1999.

Propensity Quintile/Gender	Year of Birth					
	1990–1992			1996–1999		
	Number of Children 12–23 Months	% Not Fully Vaccinated	OR¹ (95% CI²)	Number of Children 12–23 Months	% Not Fully Vaccinated	OR¹ (95% CI²)
Overall:						
Male	5,605	65.4%	1.12 (1.02–1.24)*	4,658	57.3%	1.09 (0.98–1.21)
Female	5,278	67.9%		4,239	59.5%	
Q1:						
Male	1,555	71.8%	0.96 (0.81–1.15)	1,027	63.8%	1.12 (0.90–1.40)
Female	1,535	71.1%		1,068	66.4%	
Q2:						
Male	1,167	63.4%	1.13 (0.93–1.37)	672	59.0%	0.83 (0.64–1.07)
Female	1,140	66.1%		638	54.4%	
Q3:						
Male	1,080	61.6%	1.09 (0.87–1.38)	454	65.4%	0.99 (0.71–1.38)
Female	941	63.7%		420	65.1%	
Q4:						
Male	1,114	64.7%	1.40 (1.12–1.75)**	847	63.7%	0.87 (0.68–1.11)
Female	1,038	72.0%		788	60.4%	
Q5:						
Male	642	50.1%	1.26 (0.92–1.71)	1,635	43.7%	1.36 (1.13–1.64)**
Female	551	55.8%		1,301	51.4%	

¹OR = odds ratio. ²CI = confidence interval.
*p < 0.05. **p < 0.01. ***p < 0.001.

girls and boys had equivalent rates of vaccination in the early 1990s (OR 0.96, 95% CI 0.81–1.15), but by the late 1990s, girls had a nonsignificant excess of incomplete vaccination (OR 1.12, 95% CI 0.90–1.40). In the highest propensity quintile, girls had a nonsignificant 26% excess of incomplete vaccination in the early 1990s (OR 1.26, 95% CI 0.92–1.71), which increased over time to a statistically significant 36% excess (OR 1.36, 95% CI 1.13–1.64). In contrast, girls in the 4th propensity quintile were 40% more likely to be unvaccinated in the early 1990s (OR 1.40, 95% CI 1.12–1.75), but by the late 1990s, their vaccination levels did not differ from boys (OR 0.87, 95% CI 0.68–1.11).

Figure 7.1 shows the graphs of preventive care for girls and boys by propensity quintile for the early 1990s (NFHS-1) and the late 1990s (NFHS-2). An analysis of the difference in the area under these curves is shown in Table 7.5. Over the course of the 1990s, the absolute gender difference went from a female excess of lack of vaccination to a male excess. The proportion of the absolute difference in the area under the preventive care curves that fell into the upper propensity quintiles increased over time from 45% to 72%, rather than decreasing over time, as would be expected if girls born into families most likely to sex select for boys were treating those girls that were born as wanted and valued. This is consistent with the contingency table analysis that found an increase in the relative gender differential over time among those in the highest propensity quintile.

Table 7.6 displays the multilevel logistic regression analysis of the probability of being not fully vaccinated. Lack of complete vaccination was less likely for children in the late 1990s compared to the early 1990s (AOR 0.82, 95% CI 0.75–0.90), reflecting improved immunization coverage over time. Higher birth

Figure 7.1. Not fully immunized by year of birth, propensity score quintile, and gender.

NFHS-1

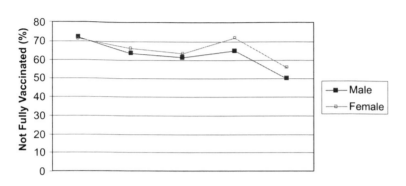

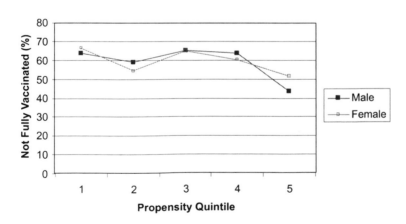

Table 7.5. Preventive care: Area under the curve by year of birth and propensity score.

Year of Birth	Propensity	AUC Male	AUC Female	Difference Female-Male	% of Total
1990–1992					
	Q1–Q2	67.6	68.6	1.0	6.8%
	Q2–Q3	62.5	64.9	2.4	16.4%
	Q3–Q4	63.2	67.9	4.7	32.2%
	Q4–Q5	57.4	63.9	6.5	44.5%
	Total			14.6	
1996–1999					
	Q1–Q2	61.4	60.4	–1.0	–32.8%
	Q2–Q3	62.2	59.8	–2.5	–80.3%
	Q3–Q4	64.6	62.8	–1.8	–59.0%
	Q4–Q5	53.7	55.9	2.2	72.1%
	Total			–3.1	

orders were more likely to not be fully vaccinated, furthermore, the risk increased within a birth order as the number of surviving older brothers increased. Third births with no older brothers or one older brother had a 22% increased risk of not being fully vaccinated (AOR 1.22, 95% CI 1.09–1.36), but for those with two older brothers, the risk increased to 43% (AOR 1.43, 95% CI 1.15–1.77). Similarly, fourth- and higher order births with no or only one older brother had a 47% increased risk (AOR 1.47, 95% CI 1.30–1.67), but the risk increased to 90% if they had two or more older brothers (AOR 1.90, 95% CI 1.63–2.21). Multiple births were independently associated with lack of full vaccination (AOR 1.89, 95% CI 1.33–2.68).

After adjusting for the other factors in the model, teenaged mothers were the only age group more likely to have unvaccinated children than mothers 20–24 years of age (AOR 1.21, 95% CI 1.10–1.34). Mothers 25–29, and 30–34 years of age were significantly less likely to have unvaccinated children (AOR 0.85 for both age groups). Muslim children were more likely to be unvaccinated (AOR 1.48, 95% CI 1.31–1.69), a phenomenon well-known in this and other countries. Children of scheduled tribes were 28% more likely to be unvaccinated (AOR 1.28, 95% CI 1.11–1.47).

The gradient by household standard of living remained in the adjusted analysis, with adjusted odds ratios declining from 1.0 in the low standard of living group to 0.79 (95% CI 0.69–0.89) in the middle standard of living group to a low of 0.61 (95% CI 0.52–0.71) in the high standard of living group. A similar gradient was observed for father's level of education, with odds ratios declining from 1.0 among children of illiterate fathers to 0.62 (95% CI 0.55–0.70) among children of high-school-educated

Table 7.6. Preventive care: Coefficient estimates from logistic regression model of lack of full vaccination, main effects and interactions.

Fixed Effects	Coefficient	(SE[1])	AOR[2] (95% CI[3])
Female Gender (vs. Male)	−0.041	(0.085)	(see interactions)
Year of Birth (vs. 1990–1992 [NFHS-1])			
1996–1999 (NFHS-2)	−0.198	(0.046)	0.82 (0.75–0.90)
Family Composition (vs. Birth Order 1 or 2):			
Birth Order 3/Surviving Older Brothers:			
None or One	0.200	(0.057)	1.22 (1.09–1.36)
Two	0.358	(0.109)	1.43 (1.15–1.77)
Birth Order 4+/Surviving Older Brothers:			
None or One	0.387	(0.065)	1.47 (1.30–1.67)
Two or More	0.642	(0.078)	1.90 (1.63–2.21)
Multiple Births	0.637	(0.178)	1.89 (1.33–2.68)
Mother's Age at Time of Birth (vs. 20–24):			
<20	0.194	(0.052)	1.21 (1.10–1.34)
25–29	−0.166	(0.050)	0.85 (0.77–0.94)
30–34	−0.161	(0.072)	0.85 (0.74–0.98)
35+	−0.135	(0.102)	0.87 (0.72–1.07)

(continued)

Table 7.6. Preventive care: Coefficient estimates from logistic regression model of lack of full vaccination, main effects and interactions. (continued)

Fixed Effects	Coefficient	(SE¹)	AOR² (95% CI³)
Propensity Score (vs. Q2 = 1.037–1.066):			
Q1 = SRB 0.898–1.037			(see interactions)
Q3 = SRB 1.066–1.088	–0.037	(0.082)	
Q4 = SRB 1.088–1.119	–0.049	(0.091)	
Q5 = SRB 1.119–1.364	–0.087	(0.087)	
	–0.173	(0.090)	
Religion (vs. Hindu):			
Muslim	0.395	(0.065)	1.48 (1.31–1.69)
Christian/Other	–0.103	(0.073)	0.90 (0.78–1.04)
Scheduled Caste/Tribe (vs. Neither):			
Scheduled Caste	0.101	(0.055)	1.11 (0.99–1.23)
Scheduled Tribe	0.247	(0.072)	1.28 (1.11–1.47)
Household Standard of Living (vs. Low):			
Lower Middle	–0.152	(0.063)	0.86 (0.76–0.97)
Middle	–0.241	(0.064)	0.79 (0.69–0.89)
Higher Middle	–0.371	(0.066)	0.69 (0.61–0.79)
High	–0.494	(0.078)	0.61 (0.52–0.71)

Mother's Education (vs. Illiterate):			
Less Than Middle School	−0.392	(0.052)	0.68 (0.61–0.75)
Middle School	−0.541	(0.071)	0.58 (0.51–0.67)
High School+	−0.721	(0.077)	0.49 (0.42–0.57)
Father's Education (vs. Illiterate):			
Less Than Middle School	−0.320	(0.053)	0.73 (0.65–0.81)
Middle School	−0.452	(0.064)	0.64 (0.56–0.72)
High School+	−0.482	(0.063)	0.62 (0.55–0.70)
Media Exposure	−0.098	(0.025)	0.91 (0.86–0.95)
Region (vs. Region 6 - South):			
Region 1: North	0.196	(0.080)	1.22 (1.04–1.42)
Region 2: West	−0.097	(0.080)	0.91 (0.78–1.06)
Region 3: Central	1.631	(0.070)	5.11 (4.45–5.86)
Region 4: East	0.563	(0.087)	1.76 (1.48–2.08)
Region 5: Northeast	1.264	(0.090)	3.54 (2.97–4.22)
Clinic in Place of Residence	−0.122	(0.059)	0.89 (0.79–0.99)
Nearest Town to Place of Residence (vs. <15 km)			
15 km or More	0.161	(0.053)	1.17 (1.06–1.30)
No Television in Village	0.295	(0.087)	1.34 (1.13–1.59)

(continued)

Table 7.6. Preventive care: Coefficient estimates from logistic regression model of lack of full vaccination, main effects and interactions. (continued)

Fixed Effects	Coefficient	(SE[1])	AOR[2] (95% CI[3])
Urban Residence (vs. Rural)	0.036	(0.066)	1.04 (0.91–1.18)
Interactions			
Gender * Propensity Score			
Female * Q1 (Low)	0.174	(0.112)	1.14 (0.99–1.32)
Female * Q2	—	—	0.96 (0.81–1.13)
Female * Q3	0.161	(0.130)	1.13 (0.93–1.36)
Female * Q4	0.135	(0.119)	1.10 (0.93–1.29)
Female * Q5 (High)	0.346	(0.115)	1.36 (1.17–1.57)
Random Effects	Variance	(SE)	
Residual Variance Between PSUs (τ_{00})	0.516	(0.041)	—

Note. Residual variance between PSUs ($\tau 00$) with no covariates in the model: 0.952 (0.041). [1]SE = standard error. [2]AOR = adjusted odds ratio. [3]CI = confidence interval.

fathers. An even steeper decline was found for mother's level of education, with adjusted odds ratios declining from 1.0 for children of illiterate mothers to 0.49 (95% CI 0.42–0.57) among children of high-school-educated mothers. Mother's media exposure was independently associated with lower levels of incomplete vaccination (AOR 0.91, 95% CI 0.86–0.95).

Children residing in the Central region of India were 5 times more likely to be unvaccinated than those in South India (AOR 5.11, 95% CI 4.45–5.86), whereas those in the Northeast were 3.5 times more likely to be unvaccinated (AOR 3.54, 95% CI 2.97–4.22). The Eastern region (AOR 1.76, 95% CI 1.48–2.08) and the North (AOR 1.22, 95% CI 1.04–1.42) also had significantly elevated levels of unvaccinated children. PSUs that had a medical clinic were less likely to have unvaccinated children (AOR 0.89, 95% CI 0.79–0.99), whereas those that were located more than 15 kilometers (the two upper quintiles of the distribution) from a town were more likely to have unvaccinated children (AOR 1.17, 95% CI 1.06–1.30). Not having a television in the village was associated with higher levels of unvaccinated children (AOR 1.34, 95% CI 1.13–1.59), which most likely is a marker for a generally low level of village infrastructure.

The only statistically significant interaction between covariates in the model was between gender and the propensity quintile. A significant and positively signed interaction term was found between gender and Q5, the highest propensity score quintile. Thus, the adjusted odds ratio for girls versus boys differed by the propensity score. Only girls in the highest propensity quintile were significantly more likely to be unvaccinated than boys. Girls in Q5 were 36% more likely to be unvaccinated than boys in the same propensity quintile (AOR 1.36, 95%

CI 1.17–1.57). This indicates that there is an additive effect of sex-selective abortion of female fetuses and postnatal preventive care. Girls born in the group most likely to be practicing prenatal sex selection of males are not receiving an equivalent level of preventive care that boys receive. They are receiving worse preventive care relative to boys than are other girls. This finding is contrary to what would be expected if the substitution hypothesis were in fact correct for the Indian situation.

CURATIVE CARE

Curative care was measured as the percentage of children under the age of 3 years with diarrhea or acute respiratory infection in the 2 weeks prior to the interview who did not receive any medical treatment for their illnesses.

Child-Level Characteristics

As shown in Table 7.7, 38.1% of ill children received no medical treatment. This proportion was higher for girls, 41.2% of whom received no treatment, compared to 35.5% of boys ($p < 0.001$). There was no difference over time from the early to the late 1990s in the proportion treated ($p = 0.12$). Infants were the least likely to receive medical treatment (40.9%) compared to children 12–23 months of age (35.4%) and to children 24–35 months of age (37.9%) ($p < 0.001$). A higher proportion of multiple births were untreated (51.3%) compared to singleton births (38.0%) ($p = 0.03$). The percentage of untreated children increased proportionately with mother's age ($p < 0.001$). Thirty-six percent of teen mothers, 39% of 25- to 29-year-old mothers, and 46% of mothers 35 years and older did not take their ill child for treatment.

Table 7.7. Curative care by child-level characteristics.

Characteristic	Number of Children	% Not Treated	p-value
Overall	14,465	38.1%	—
Gender:			
Male	7,856	35.5%	
Female	6,609	41.2%	<0.001
Year of Birth:			
1990–1992 (NFHS-1)	5,373	37.0%	
1996–1999 (NFHS-2)	9,092	38.8%	0.12
Age of Child:			
0–11 Months	14,073	40.9%	
12–23 Months	13,971	35.4%	
24–35 Months	13,105	37.9%	<0.001
Multiple Births:			
No	14,286	38.0%	
Yes	179	51.3%	0.03
Mother's Age at Time of Birth:			
<20	3,044	36.4%	
20–24	5,582	37.1%	
25–29	3,589	38.8%	
30–34	1,511	41.0%	
35+	739	45.9%	<0.001
Birth Order:			
1	3,926	31.5%	
2	3,519	36.9%	
3	2,613	40.2%	
4+	4,407	43.6%	<0.001

(continued)

Table 7.7. Curative care by child-level characteristics. *(continued)*

Characteristic	Number of Children	% Not Treated	p-value
Family Composition (Siblings):			
Birth Order 1	3,926	31.5%	
Birth Order 2:			
No Surviving Older Brothers	1,966	37.3%	
One Surviving Older Brother	1,553	36.3%	
Birth Order 3:			
No Surviving Older Brothers	873	39.3%	
One Surviving Older Brother	1,280	40.4%	
Two Surviving Older Brothers	460	41.0%	
Birth Order 4 or Higher:			
No Surviving Older Brothers	703	41.5%	
One Surviving Older Brothers	1,568	42.4%	
Two or More Surviving Older Brothers	2,136	45.2%	<0.001
Propensity Score (Quintiles):			
Q1 = SRB 0.898–1.037	3,796	41.5%	
Q2 = SRB 1.037–1.066	2,580	39.6%	
Q3 = SRB 1.066–1.088	1,760	37.8%	
Q4 = SRB 1.088–1.119	2,736	37.1%	
Q5 = SRB 1.119–1.364	3,487	32.1%	<0.001

The percentage untreated increased with increasing birth order from 31.5% of first births to 43.6% of fourth- and higher order births ($p < 0.001$). Within the higher birth orders, the gender composition of surviving older siblings was associated with treatment rates. Among third births, the percentage untreated increased as the number of older brothers increased from 39% of those with no older brothers to 41% of those with two older brothers, and among fourth- and higher order births, 41.5% of those with no older brothers remained untreated, whereas 45.2% of those with two or more older brothers were not treated. The percentage of children not treated for their illness declined as the propensity score quintile increased (p < 0.001). Forty-one percent of children in Q1 received no treatment, 38% of children in Q3, and 32% of children in Q5 received no treatment for their illness.

Family-Level Characteristics
As shown in Table 7.8, Christians (41%) and Hindus (39%) had the highest percentages of untreated children, followed by Muslims (35%) and those of other religions (23%) (p < 0.001).

Half of children belonging to scheduled tribes received no medical care for their illness, compared to 39% of children belonging to schedule castes, and 36% of other children (p < 0.001). The percentage of children who were not treated declined as the household standard of living increased. Forty-seven percent of children from households with a low standard of living were not treated, compared to 40% of children from households with a mid-level standard of living and 24% of children from households with a high standard of living (p < 0.001). Similarly, as parents' levels of education rose, the percentage of children not treated declined. Forty-three percent of children of illiterate mothers were not taken for medical treatment, which dropped to half that percentage for children of high-school-educated mothers (22%). Twenty-nine percent of children of fathers educated through high school or more were not treated, compared to 47% of children of illiterate fathers (p < 0.001). Employed mothers were found to have higher percentages of untreated children, regardless of whether they worked for cash or not. Forty-two

Table 7.8. Curative care by family-level characteristics.

Characteristic	Number of Children	% Not Treated	p-value
Religion:			
Hindu	10,582	39.3%	
Muslim	2,164	34.7%	
Christian	1,029	41.4%	
Other	677	22.5%	<0.001
Scheduled Caste/Tribe:			
Scheduled Caste	2,445	39.4%	
Scheduled Tribe	2,279	50.2%	
Neither	9,667	35.9%	<0.001
Household Standard of Living (Quintiles):			
Low	2,770	47.2%	
Lower Middle	2,933	43.0%	
Middle	2,954	39.6%	
Higher Middle	3,089	33.1%	
High	2,719	24.3%	<0.001
Mother's Education:			
Illiterate	8,378	43.4%	
< Middle School	2,976	33.5%	
Middle School	1,398	27.7%	
High School+	1,712	22.2%	<0.001
Father's Education:			
Illiterate	4,341	46.7%	
< Middle School	3,967	38.3%	
Middle School	2,281	33.4%	
High School+	3,820	29.2%	<0.001
Mother's Labor Force Participation:			
None	9,769	36.2%	
Noncash	2,008	41.8%	
Cash	2,682	42.6%	<0.001

(continued)

Table 7.8. Curative care by family-level characteristics. *(continued)*

Characteristic	Number of Children	% Not Treated	p-value
Mother's Residence Here Before/After Marriage:			
Lived Here Before Marriage	6,285	36.9%	
Moved Here at Marriage	5,028	38.6%	
Moved Here after Marriage	3,152	39.7%	0.09
Mother Tongue:			
Group 1	8,545	38.5%	
Group 2	645	26.3%	
Group 4	1,628	31.9%	
Other	3,645	49.8%	<0.001
Media Exposure:			
None	6,656	45.0%	
One	4,166	33.5%	
Two	2,971	29.3%	
Three	672	25.5%	<0.001

percent of noncash workers and 43% of cash earners did not take their children for treatment, compared to 36% of unemployed mothers ($p < 0.001$). The mother's residence in the current location before or after marriage was not associated with the percentage of children treated ($p = 0.09$). Native speakers of Group 2 (26%) and Group 4 (32%) languages had lower percentages of untreated ill children, compared to speakers of Group 1 (39%) and other (50%) languages ($p < 0.001$). The greater number of media sources the mother is regularly exposed to, the lower the percentage of untreated ill children ($p < 0.001$). Forty-five percent of women with no media sources, 33% of women with one media source, and 25% of women with three media sources did not take their ill children for medical treatment.

PSU-Level Characteristics

As expected, a greater percentage of rural children were not treated (41%) compared to urban residents (27%) (p < 0.001), as shown in Table 7.9. Children in the Northeast region had the highest levels of not receiving treatment (58%), followed by those in the East (47%) and Central (42%) regions. Children residing in the North had very low levels of not being treated (19%), and lower levels were observed in the West (29%) and South (32%). Lack of treatment was lower for those living in a village with a primary health center (37%) compared to 42% of children without a primary health center (p = 0.004). The presence of a mobile health unit had no association with treatment rates (p = 0.30), but the presence of a medical clinic did (p < 0.001). Thirty-four percent of ill children living in a village with a clinic received medical treatment, compared to 43% of those without a clinic. Similarly, the proximity to a hospital was associated with lower rates of children not being treated for their illness; 38% of those residing 0–3 kilometers or 4–7 kilometers from a hospital were not treated, compared to 41% of those 8–12 kilometers from a hospital and 44% of those 13–21 kilometers or 22 or more kilometers from a hospital (p < 0.001). Lack of electricity in the village and no television in the village were associated with lack of treatment. Over half of those (54%) living in a village with no television remained untreated, as did 49% of those with no electricity. Treatment was associated as well with the size of the village. Forty-eight percent of children in villages with less than 125 households did not receive treatment, compared to 36% of children in village with 745 or more households (p < 0.001).

Table 7.9. Curative care by PSU-level characteristics.

Characteristic	Number of Children	% Not Treated	p-value
Urban/Rural Residence:			
Urban	3,592	27.0%	
Rural	10,873	41.1%	<0.001
Region:			
Region 1: North	2,326	18.9%	
Region 2: West	1,381	28.5%	
Region 3: Central	5,443	41.8%	
Region 4: East	1,428	47.0%	
Region 5: Northeast	2,143	58.4%	
Region 6: South	1,744	31.8%	<0.001
Primary Health Center in Village:			
No	9,177	41.8%	
Yes	1,482	36.6%	0.004
Mobile Health Unit in Village:			
No	9,006	41.4%	
Yes	1,762	39.6%	0.30
Clinic in Village:			
No	7,989	42.6%	
Yes	2,119	33.5%	<0.001
Nearest Hospital to Village (Quintiles):			
0–3 km	2,157	37.5%	
4–7 km	2,076	38.3%	
8–12 km	1,982	41.3%	
13–21 km	1,947	44.4%	
>22 km	2,524	43.8%	0.001
Nearest Town to Village (Quintiles):			
0–5 km	2,390	36.5%	
6–9 km	1,837	42.9%	

(continued)

Table 7.9. Curative care by PSU-level characteristics. *(continued)*

Characteristic	Number of Children	% Not Treated	p-value
10–14 km	1,970	39.3%	
15–24 km	2,233	42.8%	
≥25 km	2,351	44.1%	0.001
Electricity in Village:			
No	2,009	49.4%	
Yes	8,755	38.7%	<0.001
Television in Village:			
No	1,540	54.4%	
Yes	8,999	39.4%	<0.001
Number of Households in Village (Quintiles):			
<125	2,235	47.6%	
125–248	2,153	42.1%	
249–400	2,192	40.2%	
401–744	1,879	41.1%	
745–8,930	1,933	36.5%	<0.001

Gender Differential by Propensity Score and Year of Birth

The relative difference in treatment received by girls and boys is examined in Table 7.10. Over the decade of the 1990s, the gender differential decreased from a 42% female excess of lack of treatment (OR 1.42, 95% CI 1.24–1.63) to a female excess of 20% (OR 1.20, 95% CI 1.08–1.33). This relative improvement for girls is not due, however, to a greater percentage of girls receiving treatment but to a worsening of treatment for boys in the late 1990s.

Table 7.10. Curative care by year of birth, propensity score quintile, and gender, India, 1990–1999.

	Year of Birth					
	1990–1992			1996–1999		
Propensity Quintile/ Gender	Number of Ill Children 0–35 Months	% Not Treated	OR[1] (95% CI[2])	Number of Ill Children 0–35 Months	% Not Treated	OR[1] (95% CI[2])
Overall:						
Male	2,929	33.2%		4,927	36.8%	
Female	2,444	41.4%	1.42 (1.24–1.63)***	4,165	41.1%	1.20 (1.08–1.33)***
Q1:						
Male	864	35.5%		1,128	42.7%	
Female	740	42.9%	1.37 (1.10–1.70)**	1,064	44.4%	1.07 (0.88–1.30)
Q2:						
Male	578	32.0%		761	37.3%	
Female	554	43.7%	1.65 (1.24–2.19)**	687	44.9%	1.37 (1.06–1.77)*
Q3:						
Male	483	34.2%		465	38.5%	
Female	398	36.9%	1.12 (0.80–1.59)	414	41.9%	1.15 (0.84–1.58)
Q4:						
Male	573	32.9%		941	35.9%	
Female	442	41.0%	1.42 (0.99–2.14)	780	39.3%	1.16 (0.92–1.45)
Q5:						
Male	399	23.6%		1,608	30.7%	
Female	286	34.7%	1.72 (1.09–2.72)*	1,194	35.5%	1.24 (1.01–1.52)*

[1]OR = odds ratio. [2]CI = confidence interval.
*p < 0.05. **p < 0.01. ***p < 0.001.

Thirty-three percent of boys did not receive treatment in the early 1990s, and that percentage increased to 37% in the late 1990s, whereas the percentage of girls not receiving treatment remained at 41%.

In the early 1990s, the gender differential was greatest and significantly elevated in Q5, the highest propensity quintile (OR 1.72, 95% CI 1.09–2.72), followed by Q2, which corresponds to a natural sex ratio at birth (OR 1.65, 95% CI 1.24–2.19), and by the lowest propensity quintile, Q1 (OR 1.37, 95% CI 1.10–1.70). Within each propensity score quintile, the gender differential declined over time, with the exception of Q3, where it stayed at about the same level. The gender differential remained significantly elevated in Q5 and in Q2 in the late 1990s. In the highest propensity quintile, Q5, the odds ratio declined from 1.72 to 1.24 (95% CI 1.01–1.52) over time. In Q2, it declined from 1.65 to 1.37 (95% CI 1.06–1.77). The declines in the gender differential within each propensity quintile were due to a worsening of treatment for boys—not to an improvement in treatment for girls.

Table 7.11 shows the area under the curve calculations for the curves shown in Figure 7.2. The proportion of the absolute gender difference that fell within the upper propensity quintiles declined slightly from 30.2% in the early 1990s to 23.1% in the late 1990s. This indicates that there has not been much improvement in the curative care of girls among those who are practicing sex selection of boys.

A multilevel logistic regression analysis of the probability of not being treated among children ill with acute respiratory infection or diarrhea was performed. Independent risk factors are shown in Table 7.12 and include the gender and age of the child, the family composition, religion, scheduled tribe

Table 7.11. Curative care: Area under the curve by year of birth and propensity score.

Year of Birth	Propensity	AUC Male	AUC Female	Difference Female-Male	% of Total
1990–1992					
	Q1–Q2	33.8	43.3	9.6	30.1%
	Q2–Q3	33.1	40.3	7.2	22.7%
	Q3–Q4	33.6	39.0	5.4	17.0%
	Q4–Q5	28.3	37.9	9.6	30.2%
	Total			31.8	
1996–1999					
	Q1–Q2	40.0	44.7	4.7	26.5%
	Q2–Q3	37.9	43.5	5.6	31.3%
	Q3–Q4	37.2	40.6	3.4	19.2%
	Q4–Q5	33.3	37.4	4.1	23.1%
	Total			17.8	

Figure 7.2. No medical treatment by year of birth, propensity score quintile, and gender.

NFHS-1

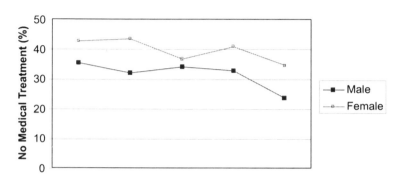

NFHS-2

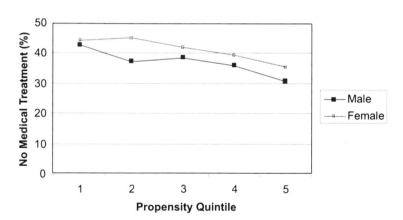

Table 7.12. Curative care: Coefficient estimates from logistic regression model of lack of medical treatment for diarrhea or ARI, main effects and interactions.

Fixed Effects	Coefficient	(SE[1])	AOR[2] (95% CI[3])
Female Gender (vs. Male)	0.202	(0.039)	1.22 (1.13–1.32)
Age of Child (vs. 0–11 Months):			
12–23 Months	−0.250	(0.045)	0.78 (0.71–0.85)
24–35 Months	−0.175	(0.049)	0.84 (0.76–0.92)
Family Composition (vs. Birth Order 1 or 2):			
Birth Order 3/Surviving Older Brothers:			
None or one	0.151	(0.058)	1.16 (1.04–1.30)
Two	0.146	(0.115)	1.16 (0.92–1.45)
Birth Order 4+/Surviving Older Brothers:			
None or one	0.147	(0.058)	1.16 (1.03–1.30)
Two or more	0.205	(0.064)	1.23 (1.08–1.39)
Propensity Score (vs. Q2 = 1.037–1.066):			
Q1 = SRB 0.898–1.037	0.016	(0.062)	1.02 (0.90–1.15)
Q3 = SRB 1.066–1.088	−0.024	(0.073)	0.98 (0.85–1.13)
Q4 = SRB 1.088–1.119	−0.066	(0.066)	0.94 (0.82–1.07)
Q5 = SRB 1.119–1.364	0.006	(0.071)	1.01 (0.87–1.16)

(continued)

Table 7.12. Curative care: Coefficient estimates from logistic regression model of lack of medical treatment for diarrhea or ARI, main effects and interactions. *(continued)*

Fixed Effects	Coefficient	(SE[1])	AOR[2] (95% CI[3])
Religion (vs. Hindu):			
Muslim	−0.236	(0.066)	0.79 (0.69–0.90)
Christian/Other	−0.149	(0.083)	0.86 (0.73–1.01)
Scheduled Caste/Tribe (vs. Neither):			
Scheduled Caste	−0.046	(0.056)	0.96 (0.86–1.06)
Scheduled Tribe	0.268	(0.069)	1.31 (1.14–1.50)
Household Standard of Living (vs. Low):			
Lower Middle	−0.079	(0.061)	0.92 (0.82–1.04)
Middle	−0.144	(0.063)	0.87 (0.77–0.98)
Higher Middle	−0.261	(0.067)	0.77 (0.68–0.88)
High	−0.347	(0.082)	0.71 (0.60–0.83)
Mother's Education (vs. Illiterate):			
Less than Middle School	−0.190	(0.056)	0.83 (0.74–0.92)
Middle School	−0.238	(0.082)	0.79 (0.67–0.92)
High School+	−0.305	(0.092)	0.74 (0.62–0.88)
Father's Education (vs. Illiterate):			
Less than Middle School	−0.108	(0.053)	0.90 (0.81–0.99)
Middle School	−0.191	(0.066)	0.83 (0.73–0.94)

		(SE)	
High School+	−0.176	(0.066)	0.84 (0.74–0.95)
Mother Tongue (vs. Group 1):			
Group 2	−0.176	(0.130)	0.84 (0.65–1.08)
Group 4	0.015	(0.174)	1.01 (0.72–1.43)
Other	0.304	(0.068)	1.35 (1.19–1.55)
Media Exposure	−0.065	(0.027)	0.94 (0.89–0.99)
Region (vs. Region 6: South):			
Region 1: North	−0.563	(0.180)	0.57 (0.40–0.81)
Region 2: West	−0.076	(0.178)	0.93 (0.65–1.31)
Region 3: Central	0.284	(0.173)	1.33 (0.95–1.87)
Region 4: East	0.323	(0.181)	1.38 (0.97–1.97)
Region 5: Northeast	0.740	(0.182)	2.10 (1.47–2.99)
Clinic in Place of Residence	−0.183	(0.060)	0.83 (0.74–0.94)
No Television in Village	0.268	(0.074)	1.31 (1.13–1.51)
Urban Residence (vs. Rural)	0.001	(0.071)	1.00 (0.87–1.15)
Random Effects	*Variance*	*(SE)*	
Residual Variance Between PSUs (τ_{00})	0.266	(0.036)	—

Note. Residual variance between PSUs (τ_{00}) with no covariates in the model: 0.480 (0.038). [1]SE = standard error. [2]AOR = adjusted odds ratio. [3]CI = confidence interval.

status, household standard of living, both mother's and father's levels of education, mother tongue, the media exposure of the mother, the geographic region of residence, the presence of a clinic in the place of residence, and living in a village that has no television.

Girls were significantly less likely to receive medical treatment when ill than were boys (AOR 1.22, 95% CI 1.13–1.32). The probability of not being treated did not vary by time over the course of the 1990s (data not shown). Children aged 12–23 months were more likely to receive treatment than infants (AOR 0.78, 95% CI 0.71–0.85), as were children aged 24–35 months (AOR 0.84, 95% CI 0.76–0.92). Among birth orders above two, the risk of not being treated was 16% higher and was 23% higher for fourth- and higher order births with two or more older brothers (AOR 1.23, 95% CI 1.08–1.39).

Muslim children were significantly less likely to remain untreated compared to Hindus (AOR 0.79, 95% CI 0.69–0.90), whereas children from scheduled tribes were significantly more likely to not be treated (AOR 1.31, 95% CI 1.14–1.50). As the level of the household standard of living increased, the odds of not receiving treatment declined relative to the lowest standard of living category. Children with a mid-level standard of living had 87% the odds of not being treated (AOR 0.87, 95% CI 0.77–0.98), those at the higher-middle level had 77% the odds of not being treated (AOR 0.77, 95% CI 0.68–0.88), and those at the upper standard of living level had 71% the odds of no treatment (AOR 0.71, 95% CI 0.60–0.83). Similarly, compared to children of illiterate mothers, children of mothers with a middle school education had 79% the odds of not being treated

(AOR 0.79, 95% CI 0.67–0.92), and children of high-school-educated mothers had 74% the odds of not being treated (AOR 0.74, 95% CI 0.62–0.88). A smaller decline in the relative odds of no treatment was observed for the father's level of education: Children of those with a middle school education had an adjusted odds ratio of 0.83, and those with a high school education had an adjusted odds ratio of 0.84, compared to children of illiterate fathers. A significantly elevated risk of not receiving treatment was found for children in families with a native tongue other than Group 1, Group 2, or Group 4, which largely includes the languages of Assamese, Sindhi, and English (AOR 1.35, 95% CI 1.19–1.55). This 35% increased risk was independent of region of residence. Mothers exposed to media sources were significantly less likely to leave their ill children untreated (AOR 0.94, 95% CI 0.89–0.99), independent of the other characteristics encompassing socioeconomic status and the level of village infrastructure

Children residing in North India were significantly less likely to remain untreated when ill than children in South India (AOR 0.57, 95% CI 0.40–0.81), whereas children in the Northeast were significantly more likely to not receive treatment (AOR 2.10, 95% CI 1.47–2.99). Having a medical clinic in the place of residence was independently associated with a decreased likelihood of not receiving treatment (AOR 0.83, 95% CI 0.74–0.94). Children living in villages lacking a single television were 31% more likely to not be treated when ill (AOR 1.31, 95% CI 1.13–1.51).

The propensity score was not independently associated with lack of treatment. No statistically significant interactions were found between the variables in the model. This indicates that the gender differential does not depend upon the level of the propensity score, nor did it change significantly over the course of the 1990s, or disproportionately so in the upper propensity quintiles. Sex-selective abortion appears to not have had any impact upon the level of curative care that girls receive when ill.

COMPOUND MORBIDITY

The presence of diarrhea or acute respiratory infection in the 2 weeks prior to interview combined with stunting or wasting is characterized in the present analysis as *compound morbidity*. Stunting is defined as height-for-age less than two standard deviations below the median, and wasting is defined as weight-for-height less than two standard deviations below the median. Overall, 15% of children under the age of 3 years were found to have compound morbidity.

Child-Level Characteristics

Table 7.13 displays the association of child-level factors with rates of compound morbidity. A slightly greater percentage of boys (15.6%) was found to have compound morbidity than the percentage of girls (14.5%) (p = 0.02). Morbidity increased over time, however, because the incidence of acute respiratory infection and diarrhea is seasonal; this is an artifact of the two surveys being conducted at different times of the year.

By age of the child, morbidity rates were highest among those 12–23 months of age (20%), compared to 14% among those 24–35 months, and 11% among infants (p < 0.001). Multiple births

Table 7.13. Compound morbidity by child-level characteristics.

Characteristic	Number of Children	% With Diarrhea/ARI and Stunted/Wasted	p-value
Overall	41,149	15.1%	—
Gender:			
Male	21,369	15.6%	
Female	19,780	14.5%	0.02
Year of Birth:			
1990–1992 (NFHS-1)	18,583	10.3%	
1996–1999 (NFHS-2)	22,566	18.9%	<0.001
Age of Child:			
0–11 Months	14,073	10.8%	
12–23 Months	13,971	20.4%	
24–35 Months	13,105	13.9%	<0.001
Multiple Births:			
No	40,747	15.1%	
Yes	402	17.4%	0.36
Mother's Age at Time of Birth:			
<20	7,614	17.9%	
20–24	15,867	14.5%	
25–29	10,785	13.7%	
30–34	4,761	14.4%	
35+	2,122	15.4%	<0.001
Birth Order:			
1	10,973	14.7%	
2	10,460	13.9%	
3	7,430	15.1%	
4+	12,286	16.3%	<0.001

(continued)

Table 7.13. Compound morbidity by child-level characteristics. *(continued)*

Characteristic	Number of Children	% With Diarrhea/ARI and Stunted/Wasted	p-value
Family Composition (Siblings):			
Birth Order 1	*10,973*	*14.7%*	
Birth Order 2:			
No Surviving Older Brothers	5,515	14.7%	
One Surviving Older Brother	4,945	13.1%	
Birth Order 3:			
No Surviving Older Brothers	2,484	15.4%	
One Surviving Older Brother	3,628	14.8%	
Two Surviving Older Brothers	1,318	15.3%	
Birth Order 4 or Higher:			
No Surviving Older Brothers	1,953	16.2%	
One Surviving Older Brothers	4,342	16.7%	
Two or More Surviving Older Brothers	5,991	16.1%	0.005
Propensity Score (Quintiles):			
Q1 = SRB 0.898–1.037	10,146	15.8%	
Q2 = SRB 1.037–1.066	7,169	14.9%	
Q3 = SRB 1.066–1.088	5,667	13.8%	
Q4 = SRB 1.088–1.119	7,830	16.3%	
Q5 = SRB 1.119–1.364	10,025	14.1%	0.002

had similar levels of morbidity as singleton births (p = 0.36). A higher percentage of children of teenaged mothers had compound morbidity (18%), followed by children of mothers 35 years and older (15.4%) (p < 0.001). Children with higher birth orders had the highest rates of morbidity, but first births had elevated rates as well. Sixteen percent of fourth- and higher order births had compound morbidity, 15.1% of third-order births, 14.7% of first births, and 13.9% of second births had compound morbidity.

This pattern is perhaps due to low birth weight among first-born children leading to chronic nutritional deficits. The rates by birth order did not vary much by the presence of older brothers. There was not a linear pattern of decrease by propensity quintile as with the other measures. Sixteen percent of children in Q1 and in Q4 were found to have compound morbidity, 15% in Q2, and 14% in both Q3 and Q5 (p = 0.002).

Family-Level Characteristics
Compound morbidity rates were higher among Hindu (15.3%) and Muslim (15.3%) families and were lower among Christians (11.9%) and children of other religions (10.1%) (p < 0.001), as shown in Table 7.14. Higher rates were found among scheduled caste children (18.4%) and scheduled tribe children (18.2%) (p < 0.001). There was a clear pattern of declining morbidity as the household standard of living increased and as the levels of mother's and father's education increased. Children in low standard of living households had a morbidity rate of 17.9%. Those in middle standard of living households had a rate of 16.3%, declining to 10.0% among those in high standard of living households (p < 0.001).

Table 7.14. Compound morbidity by family-level characteristics.

Characteristic	Number of Children	% With Diarrhea/ARI and Stunted/Wasted	p-value
Religion:			
Hindu	30,276	15.3%	
Muslim	5,612	15.3%	
Christian	3,072	11.9%	
Other	2,165	10.1%	<0.001
Scheduled Caste/Tribe:			
Scheduled Caste	6,648	18.4%	
Scheduled Tribe	5,758	18.2%	
Neither	28,611	13.8%	<0.001
Household Standard of Living (Quintiles):			
Low	6,986	17.9%	
Lower Middle	7,748	17.1%	
Middle	8,050	16.3%	
Higher Middle	9,099	14.2%	
High	9,266	10.0%	<0.001
Mother's Education:			
Illiterate	22,825	17.0%	
< Middle School	7,921	15.2%	
Middle School	4,061	11.9%	
High School+	6,338	7.8%	<0.001
Father's Education:			
Illiterate	11,562	17.4%	
< Middle School	10,456	17.0%	
Middle School	6,438	14.5%	
High School+	12,549	11.2%	<0.001
Mother's Labor Force Participation:			
None	29,362	13.6%	

(continued)

Table 7.14. Compound morbidity by family-level characteristics. *(continued)*

Characteristic	*Number of Children*	*% With Diarrhea/ARI and Stunted/Wasted*	*p-value*
Noncash	5,017	18.5%	
Cash	6,755	18.8%	<0.001
Mother's Residence Here Before/After Marriage:			
Lived Here Before Marriage	16,558	15.9%	
Moved Here at Marriage	15,683	14.0%	
Moved Here After Marriage	8,908	15.6%	<0.001
Mother Tongue:			
Group 1	24,126	15.8%	
Group 2	2,608	13.4%	
Group 4	4,733	11.6%	
Other	9,676	16.5%	<0.001
Media Exposure:			
None	18,589	16.7%	
One	11,792	14.8%	
Two	8,962	12.1%	
Three	1,806	10.2%	<0.001

Children of illiterate mothers had a high morbidity rate of 17.0%, whereas those whose mothers completed middle school had a rate of 11.9%, and children whose mothers completed high school had a very low rate of 7.8% (p < 0.001). By father's level of education, 17% of children whose father did not complete middle school were found to have compound morbidity, as were 14.5% of those whose fathers completed middle school and 11.2% of those whose fathers completed high school (p < 0.001).

Children of employed mothers had higher rates of compound morbidity: 18.5% of children of mothers not working for cash and 18.8% of children of cash earners, compared to 13.6% of children of women not working (p < 0.001). A slightly lower rate of morbidity was found for children whose mothers moved to their current place of residence at the time of marriage. Fourteen percent of children of women practicing spatial exogamy (i.e., moving out of their native place of birth for marriage) had compound morbidity, compared to 15.6% among those whose mothers moved to their current location after the time of marriage and 15.9% among those whose mothers lived in their current place of residence prior to marriage (p < 0.001). The morbidity rate decreased linearly with an increase in mother's exposure to sources of media from 16.7% among children of mothers with no regular exposure to media to 14.8% among children of those with one source to 12.1% among children of mothers with two sources to 10.2% among children of mothers with three sources of exposure to media (p < 0.001).

By native tongue, families speaking Group 4 languages had low rates of morbidity among their children (11.6%) compared to 13.4% among Group 2 language speakers, 15.8% among Group 1 language speakers, and 16.5% among native speakers of other languages (p < 0.001).

PSU-Level Characteristics

Rural areas had higher rates of compound morbidity than urban areas, 16.0% and 11.9%, respectively, as shown in Table 7.15.

Table 7.15. Compound morbidity by PSU-level characteristics.

Characteristic	Number of Children	% With Diarrhea/ARI and Stunted/Wasted	p-value
Urban/Rural Residence:			
Urban	11,668	11.9%	
Rural	29,481	16.0%	<0.001
Region:			
Region 1: North	7,078	11.5%	
Region 2: West	5,268	13.0%	
Region 3: Central	14,671	17.3%	
Region 4: East	3,174	18.0%	
Region 5: Northeast	5,832	12.6%	
Region 6: South	5,126	11.8%	<0.001
Primary Health Center in Village:			
No	24,661	16.2%	
Yes	4,163	15.4%	0.30
Mobile Health Unit in Village:			
No	24,013	16.3%	
Yes	5,131	15.0%	0.13
Clinic in Village:			
No	20,439	17.4%	
Yes	6,671	12.7%	<0.001
Nearest Hospital to Village (Quintiles):			
0–3 km	6,254	14.6%	
4–7 km	5,566	16.1%	
8–12 km	5,636	14.8%	
13–21 km	5,168	16.6%	
≥22 km	6,239	18.6%	<0.001

(continued)

Table 7.15. Compound morbidity by PSU-level characteristics. *(continued)*

Characteristic	Number of Children	% With Diarrhea/ARI and Stunted/Wasted	p-value
Nearest Town to Village (Quintiles):			
0–5 km	6,325	16.9%	
6–9 km	5,104	15.4%	
10–14 km	5,546	15.8%	
15–24 km	6,040	16.6%	
≥25 km	6,182	15.6%	0.47
Electricity in Village:			
No	5,387	18.2%	
Yes	23,699	15.5%	0.001
Television in Village:			
No	4,076	17.7%	
Yes	24,657	15.8%	0.06
Number of Households in Village (Quintiles):			
<125	5,385	16.8%	
125–248	5,975	16.9%	
249–400	5,943	16.5%	
401–744	5,020	16.8%	
745–8,930	5,564	14.7%	0.16

By region, morbidity was lowest in the North (11.5%) and South (11.8%), next lowest in the Northeast (12.6%) and West (13.0%), and highest in the Central (17.3%) and Eastern (18.0%) regions ($p < 0.001$).

Morbidity rates did not vary by the presence of a primary health center or mobile health unit but were lower in locations with a medical clinic (12.7%) (p < 0.001). Higher rates (18.6%) were found in areas that were located 22 kilometers or further from a hospital, but proximity to a town was not associated with morbidity rates (p = 0.47) nor was the size of the village in terms of the number of households (p = 0.16). Villages without electricity had an elevated rate of 18.2% (p = 0.001), and villages without any televisions had a rate of 17.7% (p = 0.06).

Gender Differential by Propensity Score and Year of Birth

Table 7.16 shows the gender differential in morbidity rates by year of birth and propensity score quintile. Girls had significantly lower morbidity than boys in the early 1990s (OR 0.83, 95% CI 0.73–0.94), but by the late 1990s, there was no difference in morbidity rates by gender (OR 0.98, 95% CI 0.91–1.06). Only in the 1st propensity quintile did girls have consistently lower rates over both time periods; among children born in the early 1990s, girls' morbidity rates were 71% of boys' rates (OR 0.71, 95% CI 0.57–0.87), and among children born in the late 1990s, girls' rates were 85% of those of boys (OR 0.85, 95% CI 0.72–1.00). In the highest propensity quintile the odds ratio for girls versus boys was not statistically significant in either time period, but the point estimate declined from 1.21 in the early 1990s to 0.87 in the late 1990s.

Analysis of the difference in the area under the female and male morbidity curves, shown in Figure 7.3, reveals an excess of male morbidity at all propensity score levels in the early 1990s, and a net excess of female morbidity in the late 1990s, but the differences are very small. The proportion of the difference in area under the curve that falls in the upper propensity scores does not change over time and is an 18% excess of male

Table 7.16. Compound morbidity by year of birth, propensity score quintile, and gender, India, 1990–1999.

Propensity Quintile/ Gender	Year of Birth					
	1990–1992			1996–1999		
	Number of Children 0–35 Months[1]	% With Compound Morbidity	OR[2] (95% CI[3])	Number of Children 0–35 Months[1]	% With Compound Morbidity	OR[2] (95% CI[3])
Overall:						
Male	9,523	11.1%		11,846	19.1%	
Female	9,060	9.4%	0.83 (0.73–0.94)**	10,720	18.8%	0.98 (0.91–1.06)
Q1:						
Male	2,422	13.2%		2,652	21.0%	
Female	2,387	9.7%	0.71 (0.57–0.87)**	2,685	18.5%	0.85 (0.72–1.00)*

Q2:						
Male	1,880	9.3%	1.19 (0.94–1.51)	1,754	19.7%	1.06 (0.88–1.28)
Female	1,891	10.9%		1,644	20.6%	
Q3:						
Male	1,821	11.2%	0.74 (0.56–0.98)*	1,125	18.0%	1.26 (0.98–1.61)
Female	1,700	8.5%		1,021	21.6%	
Q4:						
Male	1,904	11.6%	0.67 (0.49–0.90)*	2,144	20.9%	1.05 (0.89–1.23)
Female	1,800	8.0%		1,982	21.6%	
Q5:						
Male	1,388	8.0%	1.21 (0.83–1.77)	4,121	16.2%	0.87 (0.74–1.03)
Female	1,175	9.6%		3,341	14.4%	

[1]With height and weight measurements. [2]OR = odds ratio. [3]CI = confidence interval.

*p<0.05. **p<0.01. ***p<0.001.

Figure 7.3. Compound morbidity by year of birth, propensity score quintile, and gender.

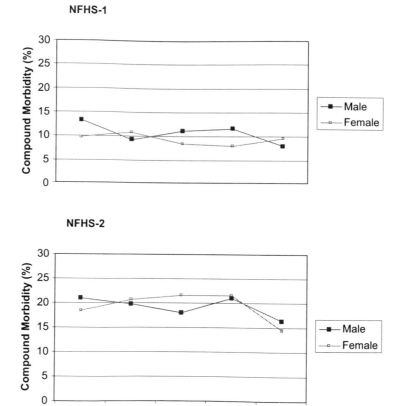

morbidity, as shown in Table 7.17. Sex-selective abortion does not appear to have had an impact upon gender differentials in child morbidity.

A multilevel logistic regression analysis of compound morbidity was carried out, with resulting coefficient estimates shown in

Table 7.17. Child morbidity: Area under the curve by year of birth and propensity score.

Year of Birth	Propensity	AUC Male	AUC Female	Difference Female-Male	% of Total
1990–1992					
	Q1–Q2	11.3	10.3	–0.9	–16.8%
	Q2–Q3	10.3	9.7	–0.6	–9.7%
	Q3–Q4	11.4	8.3	–3.2	–55.8%
	Q4–Q5	9.8	8.8	–1.0	–17.7%
	Total			–5.7	
1996–1999					
	Q1–Q2	20.4	19.6	–0.8	–26.2%
	Q2–Q3	18.9	21.1	2.3	73.8%
	Q3–Q4	19.5	21.6	2.2	70.5%
	Q4–Q5	18.6	18.0	–0.5	–18.0%
	Total			3.1	

Table 7.18. Compound morbidity: Coefficient estimates from logistic regression model, main effects and interactions.

Fixed Effects	Coefficient	(SE[1])	AOR[2] (95% CI[3])
Female Gender (vs. Male)	−0.104	(0.030)	0.90 (0.85–0.96)
Year of Birth (vs. 1990–1992 [NFHS-1]):			
1996–1999 (NFHS-2)	0.731	(0.040)	2.08 (1.92–2.25)
Age of Child (vs. 0–11 Months):			
12–23 Months	0.783	(0.038)	2.19 (2.03–2.35)
24–35 Months	0.340	(0.040)	1.40 (1.30–1.52)
Family Composition (vs. Birth Order 1 or 2):			
Birth Order 3/Surviving Older Brothers:			
None or One	0.062	(0.048)	1.06 (0.97–1.17)
Two	0.101	(0.092)	1.11 (0.92–1.33)
Birth Order 4+/Surviving Older Brothers:			
None or One	0.121	(0.054)	1.13 (1.02–1.25)
Two or More	0.161	(0.061)	1.17 (1.04–1.32)
Mother's Age at Time of Birth (vs. 20–24):			
<20	0.169	(0.044)	1.18 (1.09–1.29)
25–29	−0.170	(0.043)	0.84 (0.78–0.92)
30–34	−0.230	(0.059)	0.79 (0.71–0.89)
35+	−0.167	(0.079)	0.85 (0.73–0.99)

Propensity Score (vs. Q2 = 1.037–1.066):			
Q1 = SRB 0.898–1.037	−0.026	(0.049)	0.97 (0.88–1.07)
Q3 = SRB 1.066–1.088	−0.052	(0.057)	0.95 (0.85–1.06)
Q4 = SRB 1.088–1.119	−0.002	(0.052)	1.00 (0.90–1.11)
Q5 = SRB 1.119–1.364	0.028	(0.057)	1.03 (0.92–1.15)
Religion (vs. Hindu):			
Muslim	0.132	(0.052)	1.14 (1.03–1.26)
Christian/Other	−0.157	(0.064)	0.85 (0.75–0.97)
Scheduled Caste/Tribe (vs. Neither):			
Scheduled Caste	0.095	(0.042)	1.10 (1.01–1.20)
Scheduled Tribe	0.087	(0.056)	1.09 (0.98–1.22)
Household Standard of Living (vs. Low):			
Lower Middle	−0.019	(0.049)	0.98 (0.89–1.08)
Middle	−0.076	(0.051)	0.93 (0.84–1.02)
Higher Middle	−0.160	(0.053)	0.85 (0.77–0.95)
High	−0.391	(0.064)	0.68 (0.60–0.77)
Mother's Education (vs. Illiterate):			
Less than Middle sShool	0.097	(0.044)	1.10 (1.01–1.20)
Middle School	−0.096	(0.064)	0.91 (0.80–1.03)
High School+	−0.480	(0.074)	0.62 (0.54–0.72)

(continued)

Table 7.18. Compound morbidity: Coefficient estimates from logistic regression model, main effects and interactions. *(continued)*

Fixed Effects	Coefficient	(SE[1])	AOR[2] (95% CI[3])
Father's Education (vs. Illiterate):			
Less than Middle School	0.023	(0.041)	1.02 (0.94–1.11)
Middle School	−0.039	(0.051)	0.96 (0.87–1.06)
High School+	−0.121	(0.051)	0.89 (0.80–0.98)
Mother's Labor Force Participation (vs. None):			
Noncash	0.185	(0.048)	1.20 (1.10–1.32)
Cash	0.249	(0.042)	1.28 (1.18–1.39)
Mother's Residence Before/After Marriage *(vs. Lived in This Place Before Marriage):*			
Moved Here at Marriage	−0.022	(0.036)	0.98 (0.91–1.05)
Moved Here After Marriage	0.105	(0.042)	1.11 (1.02–1.21)

		(SE)	AOR (CI)
Region (vs. Region 6: South):			
Region 1: North	0.434	(0.072)	1.54 (1.34–1.78)
Region 2: West	0.207	(0.072)	1.23 (1.07–1.42)
Region 3: Central	0.532	(0.062)	1.70 (1.51–1.92)
Region 4: East	0.386	(0.081)	1.47 (1.26–1.72)
Region 5: Northeast	0.159	(0.078)	1.17 (1.01–1.37)
Clinic in Place of Residence	−0.131	(0.051)	0.88 (0.79–0.97)
No Television in Village	0.133	(0.061)	1.14 (1.01–1.29)
Urban Residence (vs. Rural)	0.034	(0.058)	1.03 (0.92–1.16)
Random Effects	Variance	(SE)	
Residual variance between PSUs (t_{00})	0.237	(0.025)	—

Note. Residual variance between PSUs (τ_{00}) with no covariates in the model: 0.451 (0.029).

[1]SE = standard error. [2]AOR = adjusted odds ratio. [3]CI = confidence interval.

Table 7.18. Girls were significantly less likely to have compound morbidity than boys (AOR 0.90, 95% CI 0.85–0.96). There was a significant increase in morbidity from the early 1990s to the late 1990s, an artifact of the season of the year in which the data were collected. Children aged 12–23 months were more than twice as likely to have compound morbidity than infants (AOR 2.19, 95% CI 2.03–2.35), whereas children 24–35 months of age were 40% more likely (AOR 1.40, 95% CI 1.30–1.52). Fourth- and higher order births were significantly more likely to have compound morbidity than first and second births; however the number of surviving older brothers did not modify the effect greatly. Fourth- and higher order births with zero or one older brother were 13% more likely to suffer from compound morbidity (AOR 1.13, 95% CI 1.02–1.25), whereas those with at least two older brothers were 17% more likely to suffer from compound morbidity (AOR 1.17, 95% CI 1.04–1.32).

Younger mothers were more likely to have children with compound morbidity than older mothers. Compared to mothers 20–24 years old, only children of teenaged mothers had higher levels of morbidity (AOR 1.18, 95% CI 1.09–1.29). Children of mothers 25–29 years of age, 30–34 years, and 35 years and older all had odds ratios significantly lower than 1.0, ranging from 0.79 to 0.85, compared to children of mothers 20–24 years old.

Muslims were significantly more likely to have child morbidity compared to Hindus (AOR 1.13, 95% CI 1.03–1.26), whereas Christians and children of other religions were less likely to have compound morbidity (AOR 0.85, 95% CI 0.75–0.97). Scheduled caste children were 10% more likely to have compound morbidity (AOR 1.10, 95% CI 1.01–1.20). By household standard of living, those in the higher-middle and high standard of living categories had significantly lower child morbidity rates than those in the low category, with adjusted odds ratios of 0.85 and 0.68, respectively. Rather than a gradient of risk by level of education, those with less than a middle school education were more likely to have children with compound morbidity compared to illiterate mothers (AOR 1.10, 95% CI 1.01–1.20), and only mothers with a high school education were significantly less likely to have children with morbidity (AOR 0.62, 95% CI 0.54–0.72). Children of fathers with a high school education were significantly less likely to suffer from compound morbidity than children of illiterate fathers (AOR 0.89. 95% CI 0.80–0.98).

Mothers who were employed were 20–28% more likely to have children with compound morbidity than unemployed mothers. The adjusted odds ratio for noncash workers was 1.20 (95% CI 1.10–1.32), and for women earning cash, the adjusted odds ratio was 1.28 (95% CI 1.18–1.39). Children of women who moved to their current locality after they were married were more likely to have morbidity than children of women who lived in their current locality before the time of marriage (AOR 1.11, 95% CI 1.02–1.21), perhaps reflecting poorer outcomes associated with a lack of social support garnered from long-term residence in a single locality.

All regions had elevated levels of compound morbidity compared to the South. Children residing in the central region were 70% more likely to have compound morbidity (AOR 1.70, 95% CI 1.51–1.92). Those in the North and East regions had similarly elevated risks, with adjusted odds ratios of 54% and 47%, respectively, and children in the Western and Northeastern regions had similar risks, 23% and 17%, respectively. The presence of a medical clinic was significantly associated with a decreased probability of compound morbidity (AOR 0.88, 95% CI 0.79–0.97), whereas residents of villages without any television access had an increased probability of morbidity (AOR 1.14, 95% CI 1.01–1.29).

The propensity score quintile was not significantly associated with the probability of compound morbidity, and there were no statistically significant interactions between model covariates. These findings suggest that the increasing frequency of sex-selective abortion has not had an effect upon gender disparities in compound morbidity.

SUMMARY OF FINDINGS

Preventive care was found to be disproportionately worse for girls compared to boys in the upper propensity quintile for both absolute and relative measures of gender differentials and for the unadjusted and adjusted analyses. This trend did not change significantly over the course of the 1990s as the incidence of sex-selective abortion increased. The consistency of this finding suggests that there may be an additive effect of sex selection of boys and lack of use of preventive care for girls, which increases their probability of mortality. There was no evidence that would support the substitution hypothesis.

In the unadjusted, contingency table analysis, and in the area under the curve analysis, the gender differential in curative care was found to be declining slightly over time in the highest propensity quintiles. This trend was suggestive of a pathway through which substitution of prenatal for postnatal mortality might occur. The findings did not hold up, however, in the logistic regression analysis, which adjusted for a multitude of other factors related to both the propensity score quintile and the rate of curative care. The findings, therefore, do not support either a pathway for substitution or an additive effect. There was no independent relationship between the probability of sex-selective abortion and the gender differential in rate of seeking curative care.

Similarly for compound morbidity, there was a slight trend in the unadjusted contingency table analysis toward a lessening of gender differential over time in the highest propensity quintile. There was no such trend found in the area under the curve analysis of absolute gender differentials, however. The adjusted analysis found no independent association of the propensity score quintile with the rate of compound morbidity, nor did the gender differential vary significantly by the level of the propensity score quintile. Moreover, there was not a disproportionate change over time in the gender differential among those with the highest propensity for sex selection. These findings suggest that sex-selective abortion has not had any impact upon gender differentials in compound morbidity.

CHAPTER 8

DISCUSSION
AND CONCLUSIONS

LIMITATIONS

The major threat to the internal validity of the study is *history* (Campbell & Stanley, 1963). History refers to unmeasured changes in the society at large over the study time period that are unrelated to the diffusion of sex-selective abortion but have an impact upon gender differentials in child mortality, morbidity, and health care. The study found no conclusive evidence that the increasing use of sex-selective abortion has resulted in a decline in gender disparities. That negative finding may be due to the general decline in fertility over time, resulting in an intensification of son preference. Without a control group, there is no way to determine what would have happened to the gender differential in mortality in the absence of prenatal sex selection.

It may well be that excess female child mortality would have increased over time among those with the highest propensity for sex selection, due to intensification of son preference, but the diffusion of sex-selective abortion has held it at an even level. Declining fertility in India has resulted in a shift of focus among parents toward quality of children rather than quantity. There has been greater investment in children, including their education and health care, occurring simultaneously with the spread of the technology for prenatal sex determination. This greater investment in children, in general, has led to the declines in infant and child mortality over time noted in this study.

Using data reported on a birth history to calculate the sex ratio at birth may be prone to error. There is no way to distinguish between female births that died soon after birth with both the birth and death going unreported and sex-selective abortions. The former should properly fall into the category of neonatal deaths; however, because of misreporting, they were analyzed here as nonbirths. Clark (2000) has shown that in NFHS-1, prior to the widespread availability of prenatal ultrasound, the sex ratio at birth was within the normal biological range and not correlated with sociodemographic factors, indicating that there is little systematic underreporting of female births/deaths. Similarly, the organizations implementing the surveys have found that the ratio of deaths in the first seven days to all neonatal deaths was consistently high over time, indicating that early neonatal deaths have not been seriously underreported, nor did that underreporting change substantially with the length of recall: up to 15 years (IIPS & ORC Macro, 2000). In retrospective birth histories collected in developing country settings, births tend to be displaced backward in time

(Retherford & Mishra, 2001). Moreover, in India this tendency has been found to be greater for male births than female births (Bhat, 2002; Coale & Demeny, 1967; Retherford & Roy, 2003). As a result, the sex ratio at birth is underestimated for the 5-year time period closest to the survey. Analyzing all births in the 15-year time period prior to the survey minimizes this bias.

The surveys were administered in the 1990s only to women aged 15–49; thus, the birth histories are truncated for the early time period. Women giving birth 15 years prior to the survey who were over the age of 35 are not included in the survey. Because these births to older women tend to have higher mortality, the rates may be slightly underestimated for the early time period. This bias would equally affect male and female births, so it will not have an effect on gender differentials.

A limitation of the dataset is that it contains information on proximate determinants of child mortality only for children surviving at the time of interview who were born in the 3 years prior to interview. This precludes the inclusion of these factors in the analyses of mortality. Also, it may limit the generalizability of the results of the analysis of health care and morbidity because it is restricted to children surviving at the time of the survey.

Propensity score methods assume that all covariates that are correlated with both treatment and response are included in the calculation of the propensity score. There may be unobserved variables (which randomization would take care of) that are still present and confounding the association between treatment and response, or in this study, gender and mortality. Secondly, the propensity score is a function of *pretreatment* covariates, yet many of the covariates in this study were measured well after the sex of the baby could have been selected. It is unlikely, however, that sex of the child would have subsequently influenced these covariates.

The actual *causal* effect of a baby's gender on health outcomes should be limited to the biological effects of sex, such as the increased biological vulnerability of male infants. When estimating the causal effect of gender, we are attempting to compare the expected response for an individual girl, if she would have been born as a boy, which may be problematic conceptually (Kaufman & Cooper, 2001). In addition, the nonbiological effects of gender are distal social and behavioral effects that operate through intermediates (Kaufman & Kaufman, 2001). The propensity score methods utilized in this study do not account entirely for the structured inter-relations among the distal factors and can lead to biased estimates of effect.

NEXT RESEARCH STEPS

The power of this study to detect a difference in mortality levels was limited, even with a sample size of 340,000. A trend was detected toward a declining gender disparity in postneonatal mortality over time among those with the greatest propensity to select prenatally for males. With a greater sample size, this trend might attain statistical significance. Data collection has recently begun on the third Indian NFHS survey. When the data from that survey become available, the analyses can be rerun with a 50% larger sample size, and with data on births up to 2006. In addition to increasing statistical power, it will provide an opportunity to confirm the continuation of time trends in the proportion of male births. For example, the large and sudden increase in the sex ratio at birth detected in the latter 1990s among high-school-educated women, a finding replicated by Jha et al. (2006) in a national sample of births in 1997.

The methods used in this study could be improved with additional research on multilevel log binary models. The attempt to use log binary models of male birth proportion resulted in convergence problems using the Stata *gllamm* module. MLWin software does not support log binary models, and the software was not able to run the models of male birth proportion with a logit link because the sample size was very large and the proportion was close to 0.5. If these technical problems can be resolved, the utilization of different strategies may improve the fit of the model for the proportion of male births, which would enhance study reliability.

ETHICAL CONSIDERATIONS

If the analyses presented in this study had provided evidence that prenatal sex selection was substituting for excess female infant or child mortality, it would have led to a complex ethical dilemma. On the one hand, prenatal sex selection has been characterized as *femicide*, the systematic elimination of girls from the population, by its opponents. Nevertheless, if a consequence of full enforcement of the ban on sex-selective abortion were an increase in female infanticide or an increase in the fatal neglect of older female children, then it would be difficult to support the ban from a public health perspective.

A separate ethical quandary is posed by the widespread use of sex-selective abortion in India. If one believes in reproductive choice, then is it ethical to proscribe the choice to bear sons, if that is clearly what women believe is in their best interests?

A third ethical problem deals with the issue of access to reproductive technologies. A woman in the United States would not have to rely on sex-selective abortion to control the sex composition of her offspring. She is more likely to have access to a more sophisticated preconception technique of sperm sorting. This technique is not widely available or affordable in low-income countries such as India, thus the reliance on the more crude method of second-trimester abortion.

The International Federation of Gynecology and Obstetrics recently formulated six ethical guidelines on sex selection for nonmedical purposes (Serour, 2006). First, sex selection is only justifiable on medical grounds to avoid sex-linked genetic disabilities. Second, the pre-implantation techniques of sperm sorting and embryonic cell biopsy do not require the termination of a pregnancy, but they are not ethically different from other methods employed during pregnancy because they can also result in gender discrimination. Third, professional societies must ensure that their members employ sex-selection techniques only for medical indications and do not contribute to social discrimination based on gender or sex. Fourth, professional societies should work with governments to strictly regulate sex selection in regions with imbalanced sex ratios. Fifth, *procreative liberty*, or reproductive rights warrant protection, except when the exercise of those rights result in sex discrimination; individual rights need to be balanced by the societal need to protect the equality of women and children. And finally, the sixth guideline states that regardless of the approach to nonmedical sex selection, all health professionals and their societies are obliged to advocate and promote strategies that will further gender and sex equality.

POLICY IMPLICATIONS

Because the psychological cost of prenatal discrimination is likely to be less than the psychological cost of postnatal discrimination, there are families who would opt for sex-selective abortion but never for the selective neglect of female children. For these families, sex-selective abortion *would not* have an impact upon gender differentials in child health and survival. In other words, the substitution hypothesis would not hold for these families. In families for whom postnatal discrimination is not too costly psychologically or for whom the psychological costs are outweighed by other factors such as economic costs, sex-selective abortion *would* have an impact upon gender differentials in child health and survival, that is, they would substitute prenatal selection for postnatal excess female mortality.

The analyses presented in this document provide no conclusive evidence that prenatal sex selection is substituting for female infant or child mortality. Thus, it appears that families with the option of utilizing prenatal sex selection do so, whereas other families resort to postnatal selective neglect of their excess daughters in order to achieve the desired family composition. Consequently, full enforcement of the 1994 Prenatal Diagnostic Techniques (Regulation and Prevention of Misuse) Act would not be expected to result in an increase in excess female mortality.

The medical establishment has been identified as a major barrier to enforcement of the 1994 law. Throughout India, 300 doctors have been prosecuted for violating the law, but only

4 doctors have been convicted, and just 1 doctor and his assistant have received a prison sentence. Government officials charged with enforcement say that they have received a great deal of pressure and lobbying from the medical community not to take action against ultrasonography clinic doctors who have been caught through hidden cameras divulging the sex of the fetus to the parents (Mudur, 2006). The largest number of doctors prosecuted in a single city was in the Southern city of Hyderabad, Andhra Pradesh, where a total of 18 doctors have been prosecuted. City officials have also been in the forefront of enforcement for revoking licenses and levying fines against clinics that do not conform to the law, with apparent success. In 2005 more girls were born than boys in the city of Hyderabad, a step toward reversing the decades-long trend of an increasing M:F child sex ratio (Chauhan, 2007). The state of Andhra Pradesh has also recently launched a financial incentive program, *The Girl Child Protection Scheme*, in an attempt to halt the sharp increase in the M:F child sex ratio throughout the state. The state government will give a family Rs. 1 lakh (approximately US$2,250) for every girl born after April 2002 who is the only child in the family, and Rs. 30,000 (approximately US$680) for each girl if the family stopped childbearing after having two girls. The family will receive the money once the girl reaches the age of 20, provided that she meet additional conditions designed to promote the social development of girls: she must have started school by age 5 and completed 12 years of schooling, and she must not have married under the age of 18 (Das, 2005).

   As other municipalities and states of India begin to adopt full enforcement of the law and incentive programs for girls resembling those already under way in Andhra Pradesh, the success will need to be monitored and evaluated carefully. The implementation of a reliable system for the tracking and registration of all births will prove to be an essential component of this process and of future efforts to improve the child sex ratio in India.

APPENDICES

Map A.1.1. Child sex ratio (females per 1,000 males), by district, census of India, 2001 (provisional), rural population.

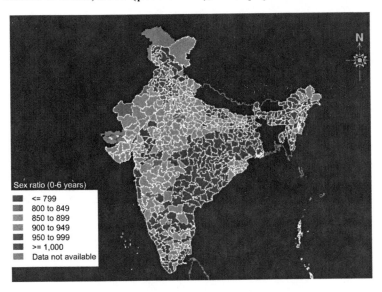

Sex ratio (0-6 years)

- <= 799
- 800 to 849
- 850 to 899
- 900 to 949
- 950 to 999
- >= 1,000
- Data not available

Source. Office of the Registrar General, India (http://www.census india.net/).

Map A.1.2. Child sex ratio (females per 1,000 males), by district, census of India, 2001 (provisional), urban population.

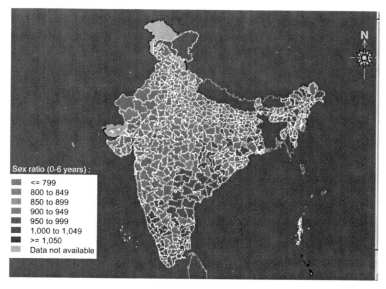

Source. Office of the Registrar General, India (http://www.census india.net/).

Figure A.1.1. Sex ratio among births in the 5 years prior to interview, India NFHS-1 (1992–1993) and NFHS-2 (1998–1999).

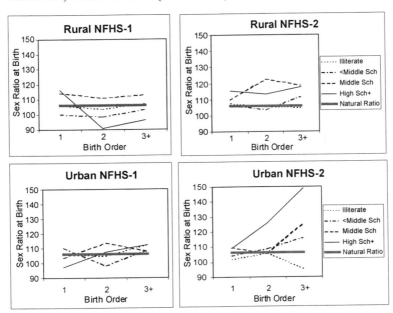

Source. National Family Health Survey (NFHS-1 and NFHS-2), International Institute for Population Sciences, Mumbai, and Macro International Inc., Calverton, MD.

Figure A.1.2. Infant mortality rates by gender and M:F ratio of rates, Indian sample registration system, 1982–2000, stratified by urban/rural residence.

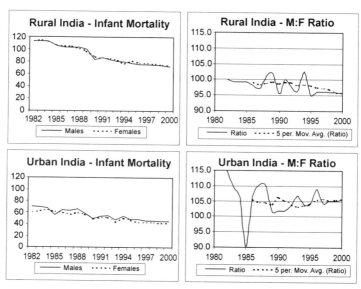

Source. Registrar General of India.

Figure A.1.3. Under-5 mortality rates by gender and M:F ratio of rates, Indian sample registration system, 1971–1996 at 5-year intervals, stratified by urban/rural residence.

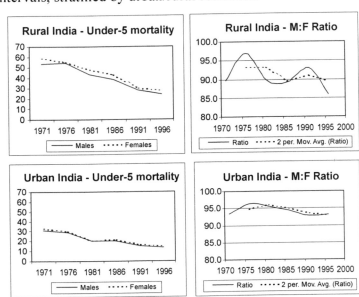

Source. Registrar General of India.

Table A.4.1. Sex ratio at birth for all births by calendar year and NFHS survey round.

Calendar Year of Birth	NFHS-1 (1992–1993)			NFHS-2 (1998–1999)			
	Length of Recall (Years)	Number of Births (275,172)	Sex Ratio	Length of Recall (Years)	Number of Births (268,877)	Sex Ratio	p-value*
1994–1999	—	—	—	0–6	59,892	108.2	—
1988–1993	0–5	61,631	106.1	4–12	75,406	107.6	0.18
1983–1987	4–10	66,585	108.1	10–17	54,107	107.2	0.44
1978–1982	9–15	57,874	106.6	15–22	42,550	109.2	0.06
1973–1977	14–20	43,777	106.1	20–27	25,591	113.2	<0.001
≤1972	19–38	45,305	111.9	25–38	11,331	113.3	0.56

*Continuity-adjusted chi-square test of proportion of male births.

Table A.4.2. Sex ratio at birth for births in the 15 years prior to interview by calendar year and NFHS survey round (sample of births to be used in the study).

| Calendar Year of Birth | NFHS-1 (1992–1993) | | | NFHS-2 (1998–1999) | | | p-value* | Both Rounds Combined |
	Length of Recall (Years)	Number of Births (185,642)	Sex Ratio	Length of Recall (Years)	Number of Births (177,004)	Sex Ratio		Sex Ratio
1994–1999	—	—	—	0–6	59,892	108.2	—	108.2
1988–1993	0–5	61,631	106.1	4–12	75,406	107.6	0.18	106.9
1983–1987	4–10	66,585	108.1	10–15	41,706	108.1	0.97	108.1
1977–1982	9–15	57,426	106.9	—	—	—	—	106.9

*Continuity-adjusted chi-square test of proportion of male births.

Table A.4.3. Variable definitions/measurement of framework.

Dependent Variables
Individual-Level (Births):
  Gender of Birth
  Survival Status at Interview, for Those Not Surviving, Age at Death (Completed Months)
  Immunization Status*
  Diarrhea 2 Week Prevalence and Treatment*
  Acute Respiratory Infection 2-Week Prevalence and Treatment*
  Nutritional Status (Wasting, Stunting)*

Independent Variables
Individual-Level (Births):
  Year of Birth
  Number of Induced Abortions in the Interval Preceding This Birth
  Length of Birth Interval Preceding This Birth
  Length of Birth Interval Following This Birth
  Birth Order (Parity)
  Number and Gender of Surviving Siblings at the Time of Birth
  Mother's Age at Time of Birth

Family-Level:

Scheduled Tribe/Scheduled Caste status

Religion

Mass Media Exposure

Father's Educational Level

Mother's Educational Level

Household Economic Status: Standard of Living Index or Assets Index

Mom's Labor Force Participation (None/cash/Noncash)

Mom's residence before marriage (spatial exogamy)

Village/Block-Level:

State

Urban/Rural

Cultural Pattern (Aryan/Dravidian/Core/Periphery, Based on Agnihotri, 1999)

Access to Medical Technology (Urban/peri-urban, Villages Within 50–75 km of Towns, Rural Areas With Well-Developed Road Infrastructure)

---

*Supplemental information on subset of surviving births in 3 years before interview.

Table A.4.4. Variables from NFHS-1 and NFHS-2 used to calculate the household asset index.

Variable and Values	NFHS-1 Variable Name and Codes	NFHS-2 Variable Name and Codes	Score
House Type:	SH031	SH49	
Pucca	1	1	4
Semi-pucca	3	2	2
Kachha	2	3	0
Toilet Facility:	HV205	HV205	
Own Flush Toilet	11	11	4
Public or Shared Flush Toilet or Own Pit Toilet	10, 12, 13, 21	10, 12, 13, 21	2
Shared or Public Pit Toilet	20, 22, 23	20, 22, 23	1
No Facility	30, 31, 40, 41	30, 31, 96	0
Source of Lighting:	SH027	SH34	
Electricity	1	1	2
Kerosene, Gas, or Oil	2, 3, 4	2, 3, 4	1
Other Source of Lighting	5	6	0
Main Fuel for Cooking:	SH030	SH37	
Electricity, Liquified Natural Gas, or Biogas	6, 7, 8	7, 8, 9	2
Coal, Charcoal, or Kerosene	3, 4, 5	4, 5, 6	1

Other Fuel	1, 2, 9	1, 2, 3	0
Source of Drinking Water:	HV201	HV201	
Pipe, Hand Pump, or Well in Residence/Yard/Plot	11, 21, 23	11, 21, 23	2
Public Tap, Hand Pump, or Well	12, 22, 24	12, 22, 24, 25, 26	1
Other Water Source	31–34, 41, 51, 61, 71	31–34, 41, 51, 96	0
Separate Room for Cooking:	SH029	SH36	
Yes	1	1	1
No	0	0	0
Ownership of Agricultural Land:	SH037 & SH038	SH44	
5 Acres or More	(SH037 + SH038) ≥5	≥5	4
2.0–4.9 Acres	(SH037 + SH038) ≥2 & <5	≥2 & <5	3
<2 Acres or Acreage Not Known	(SH037 + SH038) <2 or >995	<2 or 9,996 or 9,998	2
No Agricultural Land	SH037 = 0 & SH038 = 0	0	0
Ownership of Irrigated Land:	SH038	SH45	
Some Irrigated Land	(>0 & <995) or 996	(>0 & <9,995) or 9,996	2
No Irrigated Land	0 or 998	9,995 or 9,998	0
Ownership of Livestock:	SH039	SH46	
Owns Livestock	1	1	2
No Livestock	0	0	0

(continued)

Table A.4.4. Variables from NFHS-1 and NFHS-2 used to calculate the household asset index. (continued)

Variable and Values	NFHS-1 Variable Name and Codes	NFHS-2 Variable Name and Codes	Score
Durable Goods Ownership:			
Car or Tractor:	HV212/SH042L	HV212/SH47T	
Yes	HV212 = 1 or SH042L = 1	HV212 = 1 or SH47T = 1	4
No	HV212 = 0 & SH042L = 0	HV212 = 0 & SH47T = 0	0
Scooter/Motorcycle:	HV211	HV211	
Yes	1	1	3
No	0	0	0
Refrigerator:	HV209	HV209	
Yes	1	1	3
No	0	0	0
Television:	HV208	HV208	
Yes	1	1	2.5
No	0	0	0

Bicycle:	HV210		HV210	
Yes	1		1	2
No	0		0	0
Electric Fan:	SH042D		SH47G	
Yes	1		1	2
No	0		0	0
Radio/Transistor:	HV207		HV207	
Yes	1		1	2
No	0		0	0
Sewing Machine:	SH042A		SH47J	
Yes	1		1	2
No	0		0	0
Water Pump:	SH042O		SH47Q	
Yes	1		1	2
No	0		0	0

Table A.4.5. Linguistic groups used to define cultural pattern groups.

Language	Region	Group
Indo-Aryan Core Group:		
Hindi	All-India	1
Hindi	UP	1
Hindi	Rajasthan	1
Hindi	Himachal	1
Khari Boli	Rajasthan	1
Awadhi	UP	1
Braj Bhasha	UP	1
Kashmiri	Kashmir	1
Dogri	All-India	1
Gojri	Kashmir	1
Punjabi	All-India	1
Bhateali	Himachal	1
Bilaspuri	Himachal	1
Urdu	All-India	1
Rajasthani	Rajasthan	1
Bagri	Rajasthan	1
Dhundhari	Rajasthan	1
Harauti	Rajasthan	1
Jaipuri	Rajasthan	1
Khairari	Rajasthan	1
Marwari	Rajasthan	1
Mewari	Rajasthan	1
Mewati	Rajasthan	1
Nagarchal	Rajasthan	1
Shekhawat	Rajasthan	1
Sondwari	Rajasthan	1
Central Rajasthani Group:		
Banjari	Rajasthan	1
Lambadi	Rajasthan	1
Malwi	Rajasthan	1

(continued)

Table A.4.5. Linguistic groups used to define cultural pattern groups. *(continued)*

Language	Region	Group
Nimadi	MP	1
Gujarati	Gujarat	1
Gujaru	Maharashtra	1
Bengali	WB	1
Pahari Hindi Group:		
Kumauni	UP	2
Garhwali	UP	2
W. Pahari	Himachal	2
U. Pahari	Punjab	2
U. Pahari	Himachal	2
Eastern Hindi Group:		
Bhojpuri	Bihar	2
Khortha	Bihar	2
Magadhi	Bihar	2
Maithili	Bihar	2
E. Magadhi	Bihar	2
Sadri	Bihar	2
P. Pargani	Bihar	2
Central Hindi Group:		
Bagheli	MP	2
Ch.Garhi	MP	2
Lodhi	MP	2
Marari	MP	2
Marari	Maharashtra	2
Pardesi	Maharashtra	2
Powari	Maharashtra	2
Laria	Orissa	2
Southern Indo-Aryan:		
Saurashtra	TN	2
Kachchi	Gujarat	2

(continued)

Table A.4.5. Linguistic groups used to define cultural pattern groups. *(continued)*

Language	Region	Group
Southern Indo-Aryan:		
Marathi	Maharashtra	2
Halabi	MP	2
Parwari	MP	2
K.Marathi	Maharashtra	2
Varli	Maharashtra	2
Ahirani	Maharashtra	2
Dangi	Maharashtra	2
Oriya	Orissa	2
Bhatri	MP	2
Konkani	Maharashtra	2
Konkani	Karnataka	2
Konkani	Kerala	2
Konkani	Goa	2
Indo-Aryan (Tribal):		
Bhilli	All-India	3
Bhilli	Gujarat	3
Bhilli	MP	3
Bhilli	Maharashtra	3
Bhilli	Rajasthan	3
Barel	MP	3
Bhilali	MP	3
Bhilodi	Gujarat	3
Chodhari	Gujarat	3
Dhodia	Gujarat	3
Gamti	Gujarat	3
Kokna	Gujarat	3
Kokna	Maharashtra	3
Mawchi	Maharashtra	3
Pawri	Maharashtra	3
Wagdi	Rajasthan	3

(continued)

Table A.4.5. Linguistic groups used to define cultural pattern groups. *(continued)*

Language	Region	Group
Dravidian Group:		
Telugu	AP	4
Telugu	TN	4
Telugu	Karnataka	4
Telugu	Kerala	4
Telugu	Orissa	4
Kannada	Karnataka	4
Kannada	Kerala	4
Kannada	AP	4
Kannada	TN	4
Tulu	Karnataka	4
Tulu	Kerala	4
Malayalam	All-India	4
Tamil	TN	4
Tamil	AP	4
Tamil	Kerala	4
Tamil	Karnataka	4
Tamil	Pondi	4
Dravidian (Tribal):		
Badaga	Karnataka	5
Vadari	Maharashtra	5
Yerukala	AP	5
Dorli	MP	5
Maria	MP	5
Maria	Maharashtra	5
Gondi	AP	5
Gondi	MP	5
Gondi	Maharashtra	5
Gondi	Orissa	5
Kurukh	Assam	5
Kurukh	Bihar	5

(continued)

Table A.4.5. Linguistic groups used to define cultural pattern groups. *(continued)*

Language	Region	Group
Dravidian (Tribal):		
Kurukh	Bihar	5
Kurukh	MP	5
Kurukh	Orissa	5
Kurukh	WB	5
Kui	Orissa	5
Koya	AP	5
Koya	Orissa	5
Dhurva	MP	5
Parji	Orissa	5
Kolami	Maharashtra	5
Malto	Bihar	5
Munda Group:		
Kol	Orissa	6
Mundari	Bihar	6
Mundari	Orissa	6
Mundari	WB	6
Karmali	Bihar	6
Santali	Bihar	6
Santali	Orissa	6
Santali	WB	6
Ho	Bihar	6
Ho	Orissa	6
Kharia	MP	6
Kharia	Orissa	6
Bhumij	Bihar	6
Bhumij	Orissa	6
Korku	MP	6
Korku	Maharashtra	6
Munda	Orissa	6
Munda	WB	6

Source. Nigam (1964, as cited in Agnihotri, 1999).

ENDNOTE

1. Sex ratios are reported as the number of males per 100 females throughout this document. Reports from India, where the standard is to report the number of females per 1,000 males, have been converted.

REFERENCES

Agnihotri, S. B. (1999). *Sex ratio patterns in the Indian population: A fresh exploration.* New Delhi: Sage.

Agnihotri, S., Palmer-Jones, R., & Parikh, A. (2002). Missing women in Indian districts: A quantitative analysis. *Journal of Structural Change and Economic Dynamics, 13*(1), 284–313.

Arnold, F. (1992). Sex preference and its demographic and health implications. *International Family Planning Perspectives, 18*(3), 93–101.

Arnold, F., Rutstein, S., James, W. H., & Boklage, C. E. (1997). Sex ratio unaffected by parental age gap. *Nature, 390*, 242–243.

Arnold, F., & Roy, T. K. (2001). Vegetarian diets and the sex ratio at birth. *The Practising Midwife, 4*(10), 32–33.

Arnold, F., Kishor, S., & Roy, T. K. (2002). Sex-selective abortions in India. *Population and Development Review, 28*(4), 759–785.

Arulampalam, W., & Bhalotra, S. (2006). Sibling death clustering in India: state dependence versus unobserved heterogeneity. *Journal of the Royal Statistical Society: Series A (Statistics in Society), 169*(4), 829–848.

Astolfi, P., & Zonta, L. A. (1999). Sex ratio and parental age gap. *Human Biology, 71*(1), 135–141.

Banister, J., & Hill, K. (2004). Mortality in China. *Population Studies, 58*(1), 55–75.

Bardhan, P. K. (1974). On life and death questions. *Economic and Political Weekly, 9*(32–34), 1293–1304.

Basu, A. M. (1989). Is discrimination in food really necessary for explaining sex differentials in childhood mortality? *Population Studies, 43*(2), 193–210.

Basu, A. M. (1999). Fertility decline and increasing gender imbalance in India, including a possible South Indian turnaround. *Development and Change, 30*, 237–263.

Beasley, R. P. (2005). Nature usually favors females. *Journal of Infectious Diseases, 192*(11), 1865–1866.

Berreman, G. D. (1993). Sanskritization as female oppression in India. In B. D. Miller (Ed.), *Sex and gender hierarchies* (pp. 366–392). New York: Cambridge University Press.

Bhat, P. N. M. (2002). Completeness of India's sample registration system: An assessment using the general growth balance method. *Population Studies, 56*(2), 119–134.

Bhat, P. N. M., & Zavier, A. J. F. (2003). Fertility decline and gender bias in northern India. *Demography, 40*(4), 637–657.

Black, R. E., Morris, S. S., & Bryce J. (2003). Where and why are 10 million children dying every year? *The Lancet, 361,* 2226–2234.

Booth, B. E., & Verma, M. (1992). Decreased access to medical care for girls in Punjab, India: The roles of age, religion, and distance. *American Journal of Public Health, 82*(8), 1155–1157.

Booth, B. E., Verma, M., & Beri, R. S. (1994). Fetal sex determination in infants in Punjab, India: Correlations and implications. *BMJ, 309*(6964), 1259–1261.

Bourne, K. L., & Walker, G. M., Jr. (1991). The differential effect of mother's education on mortality of boys and girls in India. *Population Studies, 45*(2), 203–219.

Broer, K. H., Weber, D., & Kaiser, R. (1977). The frequency of Y chromatin-positive spermatozoa during in vitro penetration tests under various experimental conditions. *Fertility and Sterility, 28*(10), 1077–1081.

Cain, M. (1981). Risk and insurance: Perspectives on fertility and agrarian change in India and Bangladesh. *Population and Development Review, 7*(3), 435–474.

Cain, M. (1986). The consequences of reproductive failure: dependence, mobility, and mortality among the elderly of rural South Asia. *Population Studies, 40,* 375–388.

Caldwell, J. C., & Caldwell. P. (1990). Gender implications for survival in South Asia (Health Transition Working Paper No. 7). Canberra, Australia: NCEPH, Australian National University.

Campbell, R. B. (2001). John Graunt, John Arbuthnott, and the human sex ratio. *Human Biology, 73*(4), 605–610.

Campbell, D. T., & Stanley, J. C. (1963). *Experimental and quasi-experimental designs for research.* Chicago: Rand McNally.

Carmichael, M. (2004). No girls, please: In parts of Asia, sexism is ingrained and gender selection often means murder. *Newsweek.* Retrieved January 26, 2004, from http://www.newsweek.com/id/52879

Chen, L. C., Huq, E., & D'Souza, S. (1981). Sex bias in the family allocation of food and health care in rural Bangladesh. *Population and Development Review, 7*(1), 55–70.

Chauhan, C. (2007, September 15). For a change, girls outnumber boys. *Hindustan Times.* New Delhi. Retrieved October 22, 2007, from http://www.hindustantimes.com/StoryPage/StoryPage.aspx?id=d875da37-d113-4fbe-a9d3-b371cb2f5bf4

Clark, S. (2000). Son preference and sex composition of children: Evidence from India. *Demography, 37,* 95–107.

Claycraft, K. R. (1989). Gender-specific abortion. *The Human Life Review, 15*(2), 36–41.

Coale, A., & Demeny, P. (1967). *Methods of estimating basic demographic measures from incomplete data* (Manual IV, Population Studies, No. 43). New York: United Nations.

Cochran, W. G. (1968). The effectiveness of adjustment by subclassification in removing bias in observational studies. *Biometrics, 24,* 295–313.

Cole, S. R., & Hernan, M. A. (2002, February). Fallibility in estimating direct effects. *International Journal of Epidemiology, 31*(1), 163–165.

Das, A. (2005, October 23). Andhra opens coffers for girls. *Hindustan Times.* New Delhi.

Das Gupta, M. (1987). Selective discrimination against female children in rural Punjab, India. *Population and Development Review, 13*(1), 77–100.

Das Gupta, M. (2005). Explaining Asia's "missing women": A new look at the data. *Population and Development Review, 31*(3), 529–535.

Das Gupta, M., & Bhat, P. N. M. (1997). Fertility decline and increased manifestation of sex bias in India. *Population Studies, 51*(3), 307–315.

Dreze, J., & Khera, R. (2000). Crime, gender, and society in India: insights from homicide data. *Population and Development Review, 26*(2), 335–352.

Dyson, T. (2001). The preliminary demography of the 2001 census of India. *Population and Development Review, 27*(2), 341–356.

Dyson T., & Moore, M. (1983). On kinship structure, female autonomy, and demographic behavior in India. *Population and Development Review, 9*(1), 35–60.

European Paediatric Hepatitis C Virus Network. (2005). A significant sex—but not elective cesarean section—effect on mother-to-child transmission of hepatitis C virus infection. *The Journal of Infectious Diseases, 192*(11), 1872–1879.

Fukuda, M., Fukuda, K., Shimizu, T., & Moller, H. 1998. Decline in sex ratio at birth after Kobe earthquake. *Human Reproduction, 13*(8), 2321–2232.

Fukuda-Parr, S. (2002). *Human development report 2002: Deepening democracy in a fragmented world.* New York: Oxford University Press.

Ganatra, B., Hirve, S., & Rao, V. N. (2001, June). Sex-selective abortion: Evidence from a community-based study in Western India. *Asia-Pacific Population Journal, 16*(2), 109–124.

Goldstein, H. (2003). *Multilevel statistical models* (3rd ed.). London: Arnold.

Goodkind, D. (1996). On substituting sex preference strategies in East Asia: Does prenatal sex selection reduce postnatal discrimination? *Population and Development Review, 22*(1), 111–125.

Goodkind, D. (1999). Should prenatal sex selection be restricted? Ethical questions and their implications for research and policy. *Population Studies, 53,* 49–61.

Goody, J. (1973). Bridewealth and dowry in Africa and Eurasia. In J. Goody & S. J. Tambiah (Eds.), *Bridewealth and dowry* (pp. 1–58). New York: Cambridge University Press.

Goody, J. (1976). *Production and reproduction: A comparative study of the domestic domain.* New York: Cambridge University Press.

Gray, R. H., Simpson, J. L., Bitto, A. C., Queenan, J. T., Li, C., Kambic, R. T., et al. (1998). Sex ratio associated with timing of insemination and length of the follicular phase in planned and unplanned pregnancies during use of natural family planning. *Human Reproduction, 13*(5), 1397–1400.

Griffiths, P., Matthews, Z., Hinde, A. (2000, November). Understanding the sex ratio in India: A simulation approach. *Demography, 37*(4), 477–488.

Griffiths, P., Hinde, A., & Matthews, Z. (2001). Infant and child mortality in three culturally contrasting states of India. *Journal of Biosocial Science, 33*(4), 603–622.

Guillot, M. (2002). The dynamics of the population sex ratio in India, 1971–1996. *Population Studies, 56*(1), 51–63.

Gupta, R. P., & Attari, S. (1994). Gender bias in rural economy of MP. *Journal of Indian School of Political Economy, 6*(1), 85–93.

Harris, M. (1993). The evolution of gender hierarchies: A trial formulation. In B. D. Miller (Ed.), *Sex and gender hierarchies* (pp. 57–80). New York: Cambridge University Press.

Hill, K., & Upchurch, D. M. (1995). Gender differences in child health: Evidence from the demographic and health surveys. *Population and Development Review, 21*(1),127–151.

Hudson, P., & Buckley, R. (2000). Vegetarian diets: Are they good for pregnant women and their babies? *The Practising Midwife, 3*(7), 22–23.

International Institute for Population Sciences (IIPS), & ORC Macro. (2000). *National family health survey (NFHS-2), 1998–1999: India.* Mumbai, India: IIPS. Retrieved February 1, 2004, from http://www.nfhsindia.org/data/india/indapp.pdf

Jacob, S. (2002, July 24). Indian dismay over UN ranking. *BBC News World Edition.* London. Retrieved August 8, 2002, from http://news.bbc.co.uk/2/hi/south_asia/2149291.stm

James, W. H. (2004). Further evidence that mammalian sex ratios at birth are partially controlled by parental hormone levels around the time of conception. *Human Reproduction, 19*, 1250–1256.

Jha, P., Kumar, R., Vasa, P., Dhingra, N., Thiruchelvam, D., & Moinedden, R. (2006). Low female-to-male sex ratio of children born in India:National survey of 1.1 million households. *The Lancet, 367*, 211–218.

Kaufman, J. S., & Cooper, R. S. (2001). Commentary: Considerations for use of racial/ethnic classification in etiologic research. *American Journal of Epidemiology, 154*(4), 291–298.

Kaufman, J. S., & Kaufman, S. (2001) Assessment of structured socioeconomic effects on health. *Epidemiology, 12*(1), 157–167.

Khanna, R., Kumar, A., Vaghela, J. F., Sreenivas, V., & Puliyel, J. M. (2003, July). Community based retrospective study of sex in infant mortality in India. *BMJ, 327*(7407), 126.

Kishor, S. (1993). May God give sons to us all: Gender and child mortality in India. *American Sociological Review, 58*(2), 247–265.

Kishor S. (2002, January 10–11). *Putting India's experience in context: Population sex ratios and sex ratios at birth from the Demographic and Health Surveys.* Paper presented at the Symposium on Sex Ratio in India. Organized by International Institute for Population Sciences, Deonar, Mumbai, and Ford Foundation, New Delhi.

Kukharenko, V. I. (1973). Investigation of the prenatal sex ratio in man by the method of short-term tissue culturing. *Soviet Genetics, 7*(8), 1082–1085.

Louis, G. B., Dukic, V., Heagerty, P. J., Louis, T. A., Lynch, C. D., Ryan, L. M., et al. (2006). Analysis of repeated pregnancy outcomes. *Statistical Methods in Medical Research, 15*(2):103–26.

Manning, J. T., Anderton, R. H., & Shutt, M. (1997). Parental age gap skews child sex ratio. *Nature, 389*, 344.

Marston, C., & Cleland, J. (2003). Do unintended pregnancies carried to term lead to adverse outcomes for mother and child? An assessment in five developing countries. *Population Studies, 57*(1), 77–93.

Mast, E. E., Hwang, L. Y., Seto, D. S., Nolte, F. S., Nainan, O. V., Wurtzel, H., et al. (2005). Risk factors for perinatal transmission of hepatitis C virus (HCV) and the natural history of HCV infection acquired in infancy. *Journal of Infectious Diseases, 192*(11), 1880–1889.

Mayer, P. (1999, June). India's falling sex ratios. *Population and Development Review*, *25*(2), 323–343.

Miller, B. D. (1981). The endangered sex: Neglect of female children in rural North India. Ithaca; London: Cornell University Press.

Miller, B. D. (1989). Changing patterns of juvenile sex ratios in rural India, 1961 to 1971. *Economic and Political Weekly*, *24*(22), 1229–1236.

Mishra, V., Roy, T. K., & Retherford, R. D. (2004). Sex differentials in childhood feeding, health care, and nutritional status in India. *Population and Development Review*, *30*(2), 269–295.

Montgomery, M. R., Lloyd, C. B., Hewett, P. C., & Heuveline, P. (1997). *The consequences of imperfect fertility control for children's survival, health, and schooling* (Demographic and Health Surveys Analytical Reports No. 7). Calverton, MD: Macro International.

Morris, S. S., Black, R. E., & Tomaskovic, L. (2003). Predicting the distribution of under-five deaths by cause in countries without adequate vital registration systems. *International Journal of Epidemiology*, *32*(6), 1041–1051.

Mosley, W. H., & Chen, L. C. (1984). An analytical framework for the study of child survival in developing countries. *Population and Development Review*, *10*(Suppl 1), 25–45.

Mudur, G. (2006). Doctors in India prosecuted for sex determination, but few convicted. *BMJ*, *332*(7536), 257.

Murthi, M., Guio, A.C., & Dreze, J. (1995, December). Mortality, fertility, and gender bias in India: a district-level analysis. *Population and Development Review*, *21*(4), 745–782.

Oldenburg, P. (1992). Sex ratio, son preference and violence in India: A research note. *Economic and Political Weekly*, *27*(49–50), 2657–2662.

Oster, E. (2005). Hepatitis B and the case of the missing women. *Journal of Political Economy*, *113*(6), 1163–1216.

Pande, R. P. (2003). Selective gender differences in childhood nutrition and immunization in rural India: The role of siblings. *Demography*, *40*(3), 395–418.

Park, C. B., & Cho, N. H. (1995, March). Consequences of son preference in a low-fertility society: Imbalance of the sex ratio at birth in Korea. *Population and Development Review, 21*(1), 59–84.

Pearl, J. (1998, November). Graphs, causality, and structural equation models. *Sociological Methods and Research, 27*(2), 226–284.

Pearl, J. (2001). Causal inference in the health sciences: A conceptual introduction. *Health Services Outcomes Research Methodology, 2*(3–4), 189–220.

Rabe-Hesketh, S., Skrondal, A., & Pickles, A. (2002). Reliable estimation of generalized linearl mixed models using adaptive quadrature. *The Stata Journal, 2*, 1–21.

Rao, J. N. K., & Scott, A. J. (1984). On chi-squared tests for multiway contigency tables with proportions estimated from survey data. *Annals of Statistics, 12*, 46–60.

Registrar General of India. (1995). *Census Atlas, National Volume 1, 1991.* New Delhi, Census of India 1991: Part XI.

Registrar General of India. (2001). *Provisional population totals.* Census of India. New Delhi: Author.

Retherford, R. D., & Mishra, V. K. (2001). *An evaluation of recent estimates of fertility trends in India* (National Family Health Survey Subject Reports, No. 19). Mumbai: International Institute for Population Sciences; Honolulu: East-West Center.

Retherford, R. D., & Roy, T. K. (2003). *Factors affecting sex-selective abortion in India and 17 major states.* National Family Health Survey Subject Reports No. 21. Mumbai: International Institute for Population Sciences; Honolulu: East-West Center.

Robins, J. M., Hernan, M. A., & Brumback, B. (2000). Marginal structural models and causal inference in epidemiology. *Epidemiology, 11*(5), 550–560.

Rosenbaum, P. R., & Rubin, D. B. (1983) The central role of the propensity score in observational studies for causal effects. *Biometrika, 70*(1), 41–55.

Rosenzweig, M., & Schultz, T. P. (1982). Market opportunities, genetic endowment and intra family resource distribution: Child survival in rural India. *American Economic Review, 72,* 803–815.

Saadat, M. (2006). Change in sex ratio at birth in Sardasht (north west of Iran) after chemical bombardment. *Journal of Epidemiology and Community Health, 60,* 183.

Sachar, R. K., Verma J., Prakash V., Chopra A., Adlaka R., & Sofat R. (1990). Sex selective fertility control: An outrage. *The Journal of Family Welfare,* 36(2), 30–35.

Sen, A. (1981). *Poverty and famines: An essay on entitlements and deprivations.* Oxford: Clarendon Press.

Sen, A. (1985). *Commodities and capabilities.* Amsterdam: North-Holland.

Sen, A. (1990, December). More than 100 million women are missing. *New York Review of Books,* 37(20), 61–66.

Sen, A. (1992). Missing women. *BMJ,* 304(6827), 587–588.

Sen, A. (2003). Missing women—Revisited. *BMJ,* 327(7427), 1297–1298.

Serour, G. I. (2006). Ethical guidelines on sex selection for non-medical purposes. FIGO Committee for the Ethical Aspects of Human Reproduction and Women's Health. *International Journal of Gynecology and Obstetrics,* 92(3), 329–330.

Shapiro-Mendoza, C., Selwyn, B. J., Smith, D. P., & Sanderson, M. (2005). Parental pregnancy intention and early childhood stunting: Findings from Bolivia. *International Journal of Epidemiology, 34,* 387–396.

Simmons, G. B., Smucker, C., Bernstein, S., & Jensen, E. (1982). Postneonatal mortality in rural India: implications of an economic model. *Demography,* 19(3), 371–389.

Skinner, C. J. (1989). Introduction to Part A. In C. J. Skinner, D. Holt, & T. M. F. Smith (Eds.), *Analysis of Complex Surveys* (pp. 23–58). New York: John Wiley & Sons.

Smith, H. L. (2003). Some thoughts on causation as it relates to demography and population studies. *Population and Development Review,* 29(3), 349–374.

Snijders, T. A. B., & Bosker, R. J. (1999). *Multilevel analysis.* Newbury Park, CA: Sage.

Stata Corporation. (2003). *Survey data reference manual.* College Station, TX: Stata Press.

Taha, T. E., Nour, S., Kumwenda, N. I., Broadhead, R. L., Fiscus, S. A., Kafulafula, G., et al. (2005). Gender differences in perinatal HIV acquisition among African infants. *Pediatrics, 115*(2), e167–172.

United Nations. (1983). *Manual X: Indirect techniques for demographic estimation.* New York: United Nations.

United Nations Secretariat. (1998). Levels and trends of sex differentials in infant, child and under-five mortality. In JohnCleland (Ed.), *Too young to die: Genes or gender?* (pp. 84–108). New York: United Nations.

Waldron, I. (1987) Patterns and causes of excess female mortality among children in developing countries. *World Health Statistical Quarterly, 40*(3), 194–210.

Winship, C., & Morgan, S. L. 1999. The estimation of causal effects from observational data. *Annual Review of Sociology, 25,* 659–707.

Zorn, B., Sucur, V., Stare, J., & Meden-Vrtovec, H. (2002). Decline in sex ratio at birth after 10-day war in olovenia: Rief communication. *Human Reproduction, 17*(12), 3173–3177.

INDEX

acute respiratory infection, 19, 22, 54, 58, 94, 198, 208, 216
agriculture
  labor-intensive, 10
  draught-animal, 11
  rice cultivation, 10, 21
  wheat cultivation, 10
amniocentesis, 2, 16
Andhra Pradesh, 17, 70, 109, 246–247
Aryan, 11–12, 17, 42–43, 68, 86, 180–181, 262–264

births. *See* wanted births
birth order, 17, 20, 22–23, 30–31, 42, 60, 62, 87, 91, 93–94, 96–98, 105–106, 112–115, 143, 146, 149, 153, 156, 159, 164–165, 167, 170, 177, 179, 192–193, 199–200, 211, 214, 217–219, 230
breastfeeding, 22

capabilities, 33–36, 42
caste, 11–12, 26
  scheduled, 15, 64, 78, 106, 115, 163, 180, 201, 219, 234
causal modeling, 4, 7, 13–14, 242
census, 2, 9–10, 21, 249–250
China, 8, 24, 49
  one-child policy, 27–29
Christian, 15, 64–65, 69, 77, 80, 83, 99, 106–107, 115–116, 142, 144, 154, 163, 165, 180,

Christian (*continued*)
  182, 194, 201–202, 212, 219–220, 231, 234

demographic transition, 9, 25, 28
diarrheal disease, 19, 22, 30, 54, 58, 94, 198, 208, 216
differential stopping behavior, 14–15, 34, 43, 64, 76
dowry, 11, 26, 34
Dravidian, 12, 68, 86, 181, 265–266

educational attainment
  father's, 42, 53, 69, 87, 192, 215, 221
  mother's, 12–13, 15, 18, 20, 31, 79, 82–83, 88, 197
  parents', 26, 43, 78, 107, 122, 142, 158, 163, 180, 201, 214, 219, 235
electricity, 44, 70, 110, 124, 187, 204, 225
entitlements, 33–36
exogamy, 21, 26, 42, 68–69, 87, 107, 222

female literacy. *See* education
family-building strategy, 15, 20, 22, 28–29

Harris, Marvin, 11
hepatitis, 8

Printed in the United States
132650LV00006B/61/P